THE TINY BOOK OF MENTAL HEALTH SERVICES

A comprehensive summary

David S Indiaka

Contents

PREAMBLE

So you want to start working with mental health services because it is a passion you have had for a while now. You want to help people struggling with various difficulties to make them feel better by getting their needs met. Good for you! This is a bold move. Many people will not even consider it because of stereotypes they have seen on social media or stories they have they've heard portraying mental services as potentially dangerous places to work in. But you have gone through all that in your mind and managed to push your mind above these fallacies and are ready to delve into service. There is just a little problem though; 'where do I start? What in particular am I going to do? Are there safety buttons for me in case I need support?' In this tiny book, I will attempt to answer many of these questions. You may not find exact details to apply in all specific environments, but it comes in handy to know bits of general knowledge about the job and the groups of people you might find yourself working with. It is my hope that the information herein will enlighten and position you with the right mindset to make you comfortable in that application, or while attending to your first shift.

The book is meant to enlighten people seeking basic information about mental health services as clients, care givers, parents, educators or family members wondering about the services their kin is getting, or anyone else who is confused by concepts of mental health. Intimations in this booklet may be viewed as overly simplistic by some for example, explanations on mechanism of action of medication, and pathophysiology leading into symptomatology of conditions does not go into details. This is intentional to keep in line with the aim of the book which is to make things easy for almost people to understand these complex ideas. It is noteworthy that any issues mentioned associated with certain mental disorders should not be used by the reader to 'diagnose' themselves or others with mental health issues. The booklet only provides helpful suggestions that show how a combination of symptoms need to be considered by qualified clinicians before coming up with a label/diagnosis. Also found in this booklet are blue boxes with more technical language. If you find this daunting feel free to skip the boxes since that might be helpful only to medical students or professionals.

HEALTH? WHAT IS IT?

Health is a state of being where one has both physical and mental fitness needed to function optimally. There is no definite measure to determine whether someone is completely healthy or not. Instead, health is conceptualised to be on a continuum with one end being a state of perfect health, and the other extreme having premature death. At any given time, individuals move along the continuum towards one or the other end. If someone is more towards the healthy side, they are considered to be well. If a person is leaning more towards premature death side, they are considered ill. Mental health and physical health both apply themselves to this analogy.

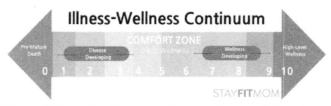

Figure 1 Shows the illness -wellness continuum. Below 5 one is ill while above 5 one is well: image courtesy of STAYFITMOM

Mental Health

The World Health Organisation defines mental health as 'a state of mental well-being that enables people to cope with the stresses of life, realize their abilities, learn, work well, and contribute to their community.' As an emphasis, mental health is not merely the 'absence of mental disorders', but rather a state in which a person can

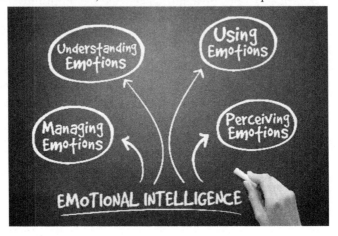

utilise all their abilities to shape the world we live in by building relationships and making their own decisions about life issues.

Worldwide, the rates of depression have increased by 49% since 1990. In 2019, it was estimated that the prevalence of depression and anxiety disorders was at about 970 million with an additional 108 million people affected by substance misuse disorders which are also classed or at least associated with mental health issues (Moitra et al., 2023). With the world population at 8.1 billion, that suggests that one in eight people were affected in 2019; yet that is not the whole list of mental health problems; you will need to add psychosis, phobias, self-harming, personality disorders, post-traumatic stress disorders (PTSD), sleep disorders, developmental, eating, sexual addiction....the list is endless.

One thing you will quickly realise is the impact of mental health on the physical wellbeing of an individual. This could be due to the actual pathophysiology (how the illness works to cause symptoms) or because of side effects from medication used to manage mental illnesses. It so happens because the core function of the brain is to regulate all other organ functions.

Negative effects of mental illness on physical health

As you will note later in the book, some mental illnesses have the nature of causing the sufferers to be paranoid about things including their own personal care. Other diseases like depression cause low energy levels and a lack of interest to do anything including nutritional intake. On the flip side, some conditions result in overindulgence to levels that vary from mild to life threatening. At times, it is not about the illness itself but the unfortunate impact of side effects from the medication that is supposed to help them cope with the symptoms of illness. Below are some negative effects of mental illnesses in no particular order.

Nutritional

Stress, anxiety and depression have marked effects on nutritional intake. While the body is struggling to balance neurotransmitters and hormone levels to manage symptoms, other body systems become collateral in this activity.

The gastrointestinal system is one of the most hard hit zones. The release of alert signals from fight or flight response shuts down most functions in this system to redirect resources to fight or run away from danger. This in turn causes loss of appetite. People who have anxiety disorders and are going through this often experience a depletion of energy sources without proper replacement which results in a poor nutritional status (Richard et al., 2022).

Depression also affects how people take in food though in a slightly different way. In some individuals, there is an increased food intake, while for others, a marked reduction is noted. Those who eat more tend to have surplus calories that are stored as fat resulting in a higher-than-normal nutritional status. Body mass index is one tool used to document nutritional status. The normal range for most people is between 18.5 to 24.9 (CDC, 2022).

Delusions likewise may cause some patients to refuse food. If this situation persists for a long time, it usually leads to a lower-than-normal nutritional status. Some medications have also been associated with increasing the appetite hence resulting in more fat deposits especially in the midsection of the body. This is referred to as central obesity. Examples are mirtazapine, olanzapine, clozapine and quetiapine. For instance, a study conducted by ? found that 94% of all patients who regularly used Olanzapine had a weight gain of over 7% in less than a year (Henderson et al., 2009).

Physical appearance and self esteem

As mentioned earlier regarding changes with nutritional status, being overweight or undernourished brings with it undesired physical appearance. Most patients end up having self-esteem issues that emanate from the weight gain caused by the treatment they receive. Other unwanted issues that come with medication include, tremors and gynecomastia (growing breasts in men).

All these factors may affect their personal view of themselves and therefore explain the self-doubt, lack of confidence, shyness, eating disorders and substance misuse sometimes seen in patients on treatment. These medications can also affect sexual function resulting in erectile dysfunction. Body image remains complex to resolve, self-motivation alongside a good therapeutic relationship can help enhance adherence to medication especially among the younger population particularly females (Lee & Jang, 2021)

Sleep disorders

Many things could result in sleep disorders including poor sleep hygiene like extreme variation in sleep times, illnesses such as migraines and incontinence, hallucinations and bad dreams, or side effects such as insomnia from antipsychotics. Depression may also increase the duration spent sleeping while anxiety may reduce sleep due to hypervigilance resulting in being easily woken from sleep.

Extrapyramidal side effects(EPS)

Brain function can be described by three processes: sensory, processing, and effector/motor. Sensory neurons bring information into the brain while motor neurons take information away from the brain to effector organs like muscles where they can cause end desired goal. Motor neurons arise from two main areas in the brain that is either the cerebrum (higher centers) or midbrain. Those that arise from the cerebrum pass through a section of the brainstem called pyramids. These carry out voluntary movements in different parts especially the limbs where there are big muscles. Because they pass through the pyramids, they are called pyramidal neurons. There are some other motor neurons that do not arise from the cerebrum and do not pass through the pyramids. These are referred to as extrapyramidal neurons. They arise from the brain stem, and their main function is to refine movements turning into smooth fine motions instead of sudden massive jerks. They also function to maintain posture and balance (Lohia & McKenzie, 2023).

Some antipsychotics (especially 1st generation antipsychotics) have the potential to affect the function of these neurons. When used for treatment, they sometimes result in severed functions of these neurons which results in a lack of control (inhibition) of the pyramidal neurons. If this happens, the patient may end up with one or several of these symptoms which are considered adverse, with the need to stop the medication immediately to prevent further damage to this system of regulatory neurons.

a) **Parkinsonism** – presence of muscle rigidity, slow movement, and tremors. It derives its name from Parkinson disease that usually presents with those symptoms. However, parkinsonism is not Parkinson's disease which is a progressive degeneration of brain cells in the substantia nigra pars compacta (Kouli et. Al 2018)

b) **Akathisia**: it is a constant feeling of restlessness with urge to tap fingers, fidget, or cross and uncross legs.

c) **Dystonia:** this refers to involuntary muscle movements that may be painful and result in an abnormal posture and gait

d) **Tardive dyskinesia**: The most severe EPS, more of a syndrome than a symptom. It includes akathisia, dystonia, buccolingual stereotypy (lip-smacking, tongue protrusion, puffing and

THE BRAIN

Of all body structure, this remains the most complex and the least understood part, yet the most essential in sustaining the body. If there was one word to describe its function, it would be co-ordination. The brain receives signals from sensory organs, processes it, determines if the information received is significant. If is deemed irrelevant or too little to necessitate a response, it is ignored, as if it never happened. However, if the information is strong/relevant enough, the brain processes it quickly and offers a response back to effector organs.

Sensory organs that first sense the information to send to the brain are to a great extent the 5 senses: touch(skin), sight(eyes), smell(nose) taste(tongue) and hearing (ears). The effector organs that receive feedback from the brain are those that can make the body to do something in form of a response, like muscles that cause movement to happen, or glands that secrete hormones to affect various processes in the body systems.

To carry out all these functions, there is one specialised cell that is fashioned to effectively assist this whole process: the nerve cell. It is found all over the body and a collection of about 86 billion of them forms the brain, each carrying out a specific function in the co-ordination function of the brain.

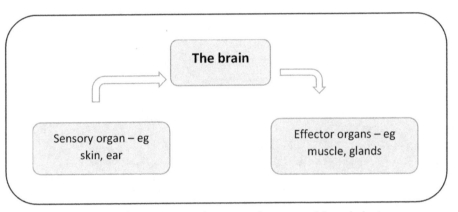

Figure 2 Figure showing input and output pathways to and from the brain

As shown above, you may think of the body's nervous system (the name given to all nerve cells networking all over the body and their supportive structures) as a computer having input signals, a central nervous system, and an output pathway.

Below is a diagram of the nerve cell; the mastermind of this entire system.

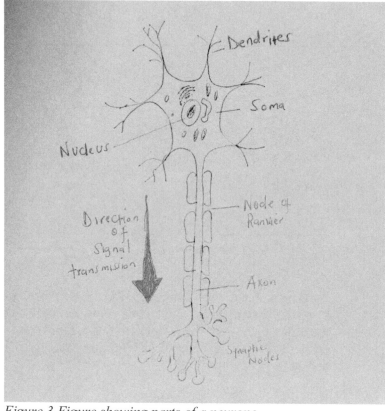

Figure 3 Figure showing parts of a neurone

As you can see, it is a very detailed cell. It has a cell body that contains most of the structures similar to other body cells but what makes it really special are the projections that emanate from the cell body. These are the extensions that pick-up information and send it to the cell body. The information is then quickly processed and passed on the tail-like elongated projection that forms the main track on which information is passed on from one nerve cell to another.

The nervous system is extensive, the brain is the main structure protected by the skull bones. At the base of the skull, it sends a long extension of itself down the backbone (also called vertebral bones) all the way to the sacrum. This extension forms the central gridline of the entire nervous system. Nerves from all pasts of the body bringing in sensory data all docks at the spine and pass the information to relay nerves that run all the way up to the brain to deliver the special message.

When the brain has a suitable response, it also uses the same central line(the spine) to send feedback to the necessary effector parts. You can see on this sketch that the green arrows showing ascending sensory data and the red arrow showing the feedback.

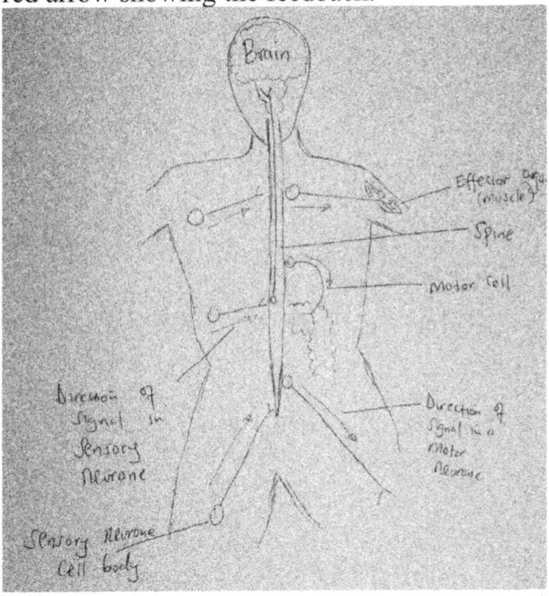

Figure 4 Drawing showing the pathways of impulses from sensory organs to the spinal cord and to the brain, and from the spial cord to effector organs

During this intense networking of nerve cells, there are junctions that exist between one cell to another. Here, information from one cell is passed on t the next. The only problem here though is that the nerve cells do not come into contact with one another, if they dis, there would be a problem with the communication process in some way. In fact, all nerve cells are heavily insulated to prevent interference of the impulse conduction process since sensations/impulses are transported with an electrical conduction system that the nerve is extremely good at.

When two nerve cells need to exchange data, one sending and the other receiving, due to the gap between them, special chemicals are used to carry out this function. The chemicals are manufactured by all the nerve cells and stored at the nerve axon terminals where the exchange is going to happen. So, the sending nerve releases the chemical, that moves though the space and the is received by the next nerve using its receptors located at that cell junction. The cell junction is referred to as synapse, the chemicals are called neurotransmitters because- you guessed it; they transmit information from one cell to another.

Neurotransmitters are broadly classified into two based on function. There are those that when released in effector organs, they result in an activity happening. If that organ is a muscle, it contracts causing movement. There are other neurotransmitters that do the opposite. Their role is to stop an action from happening. These are particularly helpful in modulating actions to reduce excessive actions from taking place. They could help in reducing the heartrate after a n exercise session that had increased it, so that the body can feel relaxed. Because of this function they are called inhibitory neurotransmitters because they inhibit, they limit, stop, or block something from happening. If you have only a little inhibitory hormone produced, then the reduction in activity will be just small. If a lot of it is produced, there will be too much inhibition happening and if this in unintended like in substance abuse involving sedatives, the vital body functions will be slowed too much to fatal levels if its not corrected quickly.

The other set of neurotransmitters explained earlier, that cause actions to take place are called excitatory neurotransmitters. They excite muscles to contract, glands to produce their contents and the heart to beat faster in times of need.

Due to the high number of nerve cells in the brain, a lot of neurotransmitters will be seen to have functions there. The spine also has synapses of both sensory and motor neurones thus has a considerable number of neurotransmitters being released and received. However, for the purpose of this discussion we will focus more on the ones in the brain.

You may think to yourself, does it mean if there's a lot of excitatory neurotransmitters released in the brain at a certain time, does it mean the person would be excited and happy? Well, the answer may not be as easy as that, but you could cautiously say yes. To an extent, excitement in real life comes from abundance of these excitatory neurones, for example when playing a game on the field, everyone is excited due to availability of excitatory neurone Adrenaline flowing all over the body. In that moment, that same hormone is also increasing the heartrate to make sure there's enough blood supply to all vital organs. On the flip side of things, the same hormone released in abundance when you encounter a scary figure in the dark causes anxiety and the feeling of wanting to flee. If this abundance is not well controlled, and that an individual is having sudden gash of adrenaline even when there's nothing exciting or frightening, symptoms of anxiety and panic will be evident in that person.

You will need to think about this analogy right here as you go through the book. You might encounter some of the neurotransmitters mentioned as associated with certain illnesses. I have listed some of the most common neurotransmitters in the brain and their known nature as either being excitatory or inhibitory and you can come back to this page as many times as you need to if you want to remind self what kind of characteristic the neurone of interest has.

Excitatory neurotransmitters	Inhibitory neurotransmitters
Glutamate	Gamma aminobutyric acid (GABA)
Acetyl choline	Endorphins
Epinephrine/adrenaline	Serotonin
Noradrenaline	Dopamine
Dopamine	Adenosine
Histamine	

PATIENT GROUPS IN MENTAL HEALTH SERVICES

Conditions are usually classed in groups in an effort to ensure that each subset gets specialist support. There are two major diagnostic tools used to classify mental health issues. The first is International statistical classification of diseases (ICD) and the second is the Diagnostic Statistical manual of Mental disorders, (DSM). Both are regularly revised by experts in the field thus you will notice new versions being released regularly. For the DSM, the most recent version is the 5th edition; usually denoted simply as **DSM-5**, while the latest ICD version is **ICD 11,** released in 2022.

The DSM is updated every 5-7 years, while the ICD is updated yearly without necessarily changing the number of the version. For instance, you may see ICD 10 having many previous minor updates from 2008, or 2010 but still retains the title ICD-10. Its classifications and codes have been adopted by the WHO and are thus used in many countries. For ease of understanding, I will loosely use the DSM-4 and also few bits of DSM-5 to show the different patient groups you may encounter in various services since it classifies these conditions in a simple way. There are 5 axes and they are briefly described below;

i)   Axis 1 : Mental health and substance misuse disorders
ii) Axis 2 : Personality disorders and mental retardation
iii) Axis 3: General medical conditions that have impact on mental health.
iv) Psychosocial and environmental issues such as loss of a job or house
v)   Global assessment of functioning

We will focus more on the first two axes as they seem to encompass most disorders. The other three axes appear to have related issues that can be considered as triggers, co-morbidities, or risk factors. For example, a sudden loss of employment is most likely to affect one's mental wellbeing regardless of whether they have an existing mental health diagnosis or not. The worry from loss of an income source brings with it additional stress that is most likely to trigger a worsening of symptoms. Also included is a brief discussion on self-harm

Axis 1 : Mood , Anxiety, Psychosis, Obsessive Compulsive Disorders, Substance Use Disorders And Eating Disorders

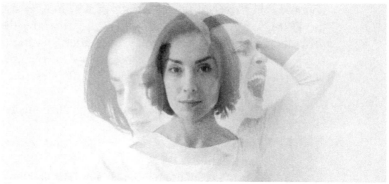

Figure 5: Image showing a woman facing ahead and behind here are two other faces fading away, showing two different emotions. One low in mood and the other upset; typical features of bipolar mood disorder: image courtesy of Shutterstock

Mood Disorders

Mood is defined as a pervasive internal state that is sustained over time and has direct impact on all aspects of the life of an including their interactions and general well-being (Sekhon & Gupta, 2023). *Pervasive* in this context is used to mean spreading extensively and so thoroughly as to be seen or felt everywhere.

Think about an individual who presents as sad all day. Some people may talk to them only minimally, some may make fun of them, while others just outrightly avoid them. Picture this as the life of the patient. Their mood has totally soaked them up. They may not like to be as they are, but that is how they are in that moment. The actions of others towards them might either worsen how they feel, or reduce the edge of their low mood. It is at this point that we come in; supporting such people to overcome these difficulties with the end goal of overcoming their current struggle.

There are a number of mood disorders including bipolar, major depression, hypomania, cyclothymic, persistent depression, disruptive mood dysregulation, and perinatal depression. I will only discuss major depression, bipolar, and perinatal depression mood disorders.

Major depression

This is a condition characterised by low mood, sleep and nutritional disturbances. The individual typically does not have any interest in activities that would usually give them pleasure.

Symptoms
- Loss of interest to do anything.
- Sleep pattern changes – sleeping too much or too little
- Changes in appetite – eating too much or too little
- Trouble concentrating
- Feeling low in energy or slowed down
- Restlessness/irritability
- Thoughts of self-harm/suicide

(Howard E. LeWine, 2022), (NHS)
Diagnosis
At least 2 weeks of above symptoms

Bipolar mood disorder

The individual has rapid changes in mood oscillating between manic and depressed episodes. Symptoms include;
Depression episode
Similar to major depression disorder above
Mania episode
- Elated feeling of excitement and joy
- High feeling of self-importance
- Easily distracted by things happening around
- Easily agitated /irritable
- Speaking rapidly
- Delusions (especially of grandeur)
- Hallucinations
- Not sleeping much
- Engaging in risky behaviour
- Overspending money without much thought to it.

(Jain & Mitra, 2023)
Diagnosis
Presence of manic symptoms that persist for **one week** or more, with irritable mood present throughout the day.

Perinatal Depression

This can be experienced either before(prenatal), during or after(post natal) delivery of a baby. It affects almost a tenth of all mothers and with it are other comorbidities correlated with it. They include hypertension, diabetes mellitus, hyperlipidaemia and strokes. It is also a leading cause in maternal suicides.

Symptoms
+ Having an overall depressed mood
+ Low energy /not wanting to do anything.
+ Severe mood swings
+ Difficulty bonding with the baby
+ A Feeling of guilt and worthlessness (from not bonding well with the baby)
+ Crying too much
+ Withdrawing self (even from family)
+ Loss of interest in sex and difficulty connecting with your partner
+ Physical symptoms that don't result from a health condition or other cause. These may include headaches, muscle aches and gastrointestinal (GI) problems
+ Problems concentrating, remembering things, reasoning or making decision
+ Thoughts of harming self or baby (recurrent in nature)
+ Sleep problems- either too much or too little
+ Appetite problems - eating too much or too little
+ Overwhelming tiredness or loss of energy
+ Anger and irritability

Diagnosis
It is differentiated from baby blues by **onset and duration.** Baby blues come after birth of the baby and usually do not persist beyond two weeks. Perinatal depression on the other hand covers a long time up to one year after the baby is born.
(Mughal et al., 2022) (Anokye et al., 2018) (Lee et al., 2022) (ClevelandClinic, 2022)

Disruptive Mood Dysregulation Disorder

This affects children and adolescents. In this condition, the children/adolescents experience intense and ongoing irritability, anger, and intense temper outbursts. They experience these emotions frequently and are noted to be more than just a bad mood. Because of these repetitive outbursts and irritability, they tend to find themselves in trouble at school and home with parents and frequent fights with friends. A child with these symptoms may often be found to be under close monitoring in school and have trouble maintaining long term friendships and in engaging in sports. The symptoms in DMDD should be severe enough to affect functioning at home, school and social settings. The age mostly affected is 6 to 10 years of age.

Symptoms
Severe temper outbursts (verbal or behavioural), on average, three or more times per week
Chronically irritable or angry mood most of the day, nearly every day

Diagnosis

Based on symptomatology and **history taking**. The outburst and irritability must be frequent; more than twice a week, and the symptoms of irritability should be sustained throughout the day. This should be seen for not less than **12 months** (Freeman et al., 2016) (NIH, nd) (Chase et al., 2020)

Other types of depression

i. **Persistent depressive disorder (dysthymia)-** it's a milder but long lasting form of depression.

ii. **Cyclothymic-** this is a milder form of bipolar disorder with the person having times of depressed mood and elated mood, but severity does not match bipolar mood disorder

iii. **Seasonal affective disorder-** a type od depression that appears on a certain season of the year, mainly winter which has shorter day periods of light. Shorter daylight is thought to result in changes in chemical components in the brain resulting in depressed mood.

(JohnsHopkinsMedicine, nd),

Anxiety Disorders

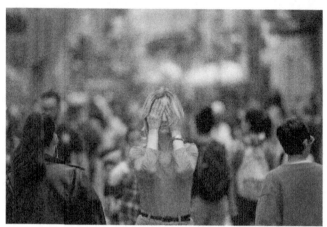

Figure 6: A woman covering her face when having a panic attack in a public space: image courtesy of Shutterstock

Any anxiety disorder will have features of extreme worry that end up interfering with the ability of the person to carry out daily activities, relate with other people, or work. These include Generalised anxiety disorders (GAD), panic disorders, social anxiety, and phobias. Herein, GAD, Panic and Phobia disorders have been highlighted.

Generalised anxiety disorder (GAD)

This is a condition that causes the sufferer to feel excessive anxiety to a level of impacting their ability to function , work, or relationships. The worry usually is unrealistic

Symptoms

- Excessive sweating

- Dry mouth
- Trouble falling or staying asleep.
- Being unable to relax
- Trembling or tense muscles
- Headaches
- Easily irritable
- Palpitations
- Trouble breathing
- Nausea
- Urinating often
- Feeling a lump in the throat
- Fatigue

Diagnosis

Symptoms are usually persistent for more than **6 months** and cause marked difficulty in conducting daily tasks, work or relationships.

(da Silva et al., 2020) (Wittchen, 2002)

Panic disorders

(Differs from GAD by how it occurs in episodes that are on and off unlike GAD that is pervasive/persistent

Symptoms
- An overwhelming sense of fear and anxiety
- Fear of death or impending doom
- Palpitations
- Sweating
- Trembling
- Troubled breathing or chest pain
- Dizziness
- nausea

Diagnosis

Repeated attacks within a **one-month** period. The attacks should not be associated by any triggers/ random with no apparent cause.
(Eide et al., 2023) (Forstner et al., 2019)(NHS)

Phobias

These are persistent and intense fear of a particular objects, person, situation, or activity. They differ with panic attacks based on the cause or trigger such that this case has a particular thing that's causing the anxiety. Symptoms are similar to panic attacks but are isolated and tend to happen when the individual is exposed or thinks about the object of their fears.

Examples of common phobias in alphabetical order are;
i. Acrophobia: fear of heights
ii. Aerophobia: fear of flying
iii. Agoraphobia :fear of open spaces or crowds
iv. Ancraophobia: fear of wind
v. Aquaphobia: fear of water
vi. Atelophobia: fear of imperfection
vii. Autophobia: fear of being alone
viii. Dentophobia: fear of going to the dentist
ix. Gamophobia: fear of marriage
x. Glossophobia: fear of public speaking
xi. Iatrophobia: fear of doctors
xii. Mysophobia:fear of germs and dirt
xiii. Nyctophobia: fear of darkness
xiv. Plutophobia: fear of money
xv. Scopophobia: fear of being stared at
xvi. Zoophobia: fear of animals

Diagnosis

The fear has to be interrupting daily activities, relationships and social wellbeing and be persistent for over **6 months** for the diagnosis to be made.
(Eaton et al., 2018) (Moore, 2022) (Pelek, 2022)

Support for Phobias

- Cognitive Behavioural Therapy (CBT)
- Eye Movement Desensitization and Reprocessing Therapy (EMDR)
- Exposure Therapy
- Systematic Desensitization
- Applied Muscle Tension (AMT)
- Psychoeducation
- Haptotherapy

Post Traumatic Stress Disorder (PTSD)

This is a group of symptoms that develop after a traumatic event causing anxiety to the sufferer.

Symptoms

- Flashbacks of traumatic events
- Nightmares
- feeling very anxious and difficulty sleeping
- Self-destructive behaviour live use of drugs
- Easily frightened
- Always being on guard for danger
- Trouble concentrating.
- Irritability, angry outbursts
- Overwhelming guilt or shame

Diagnosis

Symptoms persistent for more than **one month** and cause marked difficulty with daily tasks, work, or relationships.

Treatment options for PTSD

- Cognitive behavioural therapy

- Schema therapies
- Medical management of anxiety and sleep disorder symptoms

Support available for anxiety disorders

- Medication therapy
- Psychotherapy
- Relaxation therapies (these include deep breathing, visualization, meditation, massage, aroma therapy)

(Koenen et al., 2017)

Relaxation therapy benefits

This is probably the most significant support for all types of anxiety disorders. Learning these skills helps to manage symptoms. They also become coping mechanisms to handle situations that would cause anxiety in the future. Most of such therapies work on the principle of counteracting the actions of catecholamines by using physical body actions that reassure the mind that there is no danger thus enhancing relaxation. The techniques aim to;

- Slow the heart rate
- Lower blood pressure
- Slow down the breathing rate
- Improve digestion
- Control blood sugar levels
- Increase the blood flow to major muscles
- Reduce muscle tension and chronic pain
- Improve focus and mood

- Improve sleep quality
- Lower fatigue levels
- Reduce feelings of anger and frustration
- Boost confidence to handle problems

These techniques appear to work well when applied in conjunction with other skills like

- Positive Thinking
- Problem-solving skiills
- Managing time and priorities
- Exercising regularly
- Eating a healthy diet
- Sleeping enough
- Spending time outside
- Reaching out to supportive family and friends

(Mayoclinic, 2022)

Psychosis (Schizophrenia)

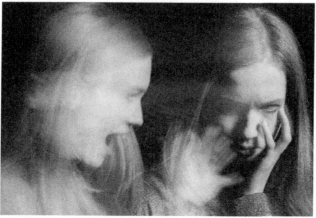

Figure 7: A girl with schizophrenia covering her ears to stop hearing the voices of her alter ego: Image courtesy of Shutterstock

Schizophrenia is a state of mind experienced by people with other mental health conditions like severe OCD, Paranoia, and schizotypal personality disorders. Individuals with psychosis have episodes where they hallucinate and have delusions. A *hallucination* is perceiving, seeing, or hearing things that other people in the same place can't see or hear. It could affect any of the 5 senses of sight, hearing, smell, taste, and touch.

A *delusion* is an impaired/fixed false belief. The belief could be about elated self-importance (grandiosity), or that the person's life is in danger (persecution), someone is in love with them (erotomaniac), or something is wrong with their bodies (Somatic)

Symptoms

Psychosis can present with either positive or negative symptoms or both.

Positive symptoms – those that are adding to the feeling or thinking of the individual. These are the delusions, hallucinations, pressured speech, and word salad.

Negative symptoms- these seem to reduce normal functionality. These are depression-like symptoms e.g., lack of pleasure in activities, being withdrawn, trouble with speech, being unkempt.

Diagnosis

It is done by assessing symptoms by a mental health professional. Other Tests may be done to rule out other causes of symptoms such as Complete Blood Count or Liver Functional Tests.

Support /treatment for mood, anxiety disorders and psychosis

These are treated with medication (such as antidepressants, anxiolytics, and antipsychotics), psychology, talking therapies, Cognitive Behavioural Therapies (CBT) and group therapies.

(Gaebel & Zielasek, 2015)(NIH)(NHS)

Obsessive compulsive disorders

These are disorders that present a pattern of unwanted thoughts and fears referred to as obsessions. They are often coupled with the urge to engage in certain behaviours, compulsions, which are irresistible in nature. When such behaviours are repetitive, they are called rituals (Subramaniam et al., 2013).

Symptoms

These may be described in the three categories namely;

A) Obsessions – this refers to unwanted, intrusive, distressing thoughts like the fear to harm self, others or get contamination, among others.

B) Emotions – this is intense anxiety and distress from thought which makes it hard to think about anything else

C) Compulsive behaviours like hand washing, hoarding items, checking if doors are shut.

Most of these thoughts are intense and behaviours repetitive. The thoughts and fears noticed in such patients do not seem to have any logical reason. OCD is differentiated from another similar condition OCPD (Obsessive Compulsive Personality Disorder) which is a personality disorder caused by intrusive thoughts that lead to compulsive behaviour. In OCPD, the individual wants to be in control and is the perfectionist in whatever they do. This is usually accompanied with a minimal disruption in their ability to engage in activities of daily living and relationships.

Support available for OCD

+ Talking therapies to reassure them and allay their anxiety
+ Medication
+ Exposure and response prevention (ERP) therapy
(Pittenger et al., 2005)

Eating Disorders

These are situations where an individual uses certain eating behaviour as a stress coping mechanism. These coping styles are usually associated with negative physical health outcomes over time. Examples include anorexia nervosa, bulimia nervosa, binge eating disorder, pica, ruminating disorder, and restrictive food intake disorder.

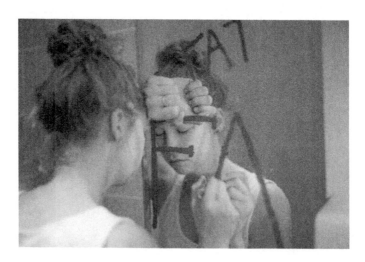

Figure 8: Bulimic girl writing FAT on the mirror; Photo curtesy of Shutterstock

Eating disorder	Common symptomatology	Diagnosis
Anorexia nervosa	• Low body mass index (BMI) • Missing meals/eating very little • The belief that you are fat (when not) • Amenorrhea in premenopausal females • Hair loss/dry skin • Light-headedness and dizziness (from lack of nutrition)	Multi-disciplinary effort. The problem is associated with social shame and thus may be undetected for long periods. Physical exam by a general doctor may hint to this problem, and then the patient may be referred to a psychiatrist or psychologist for further assessment
Bulimia nervosa	• Scars/ calluses on knuckles (from injuries caused by teeth as they try to induce vomiting with ringers inserted in the throat.) • Excessively exercising • Blood shot eyes • Hiding food to binge and purge later • Misuse of some medication such as diuretics • Frequent use of toilets	Closely shares triggers and symptoms with anorexia nervosa, but here the individual eats a large amount of food and purges to get rid of it with the aim of controlling their own weight. Multidisciplinary effort is needed to diagnose this disorder too.

Pica

This is an eating disorder that involves eating objects not considered as food such as soil, faeces, sharp objects, chewing ice or paper. Some of these objects present potential detriment to their physical health. Some individuals with iron deficiency have been seen to be affected by this eating disorder. Many objects can be involved and here are some terms used to describe various pica behaviours

- Acuphagia (Sharp Objects)
- Amylophagia (Starch)
- Cautopyreiophagia (Burnt Matches)
- Coniophagia (Dust)
- Coprophagia (Feces)
- Emetophagia (Vomit)
- Geomelophagia (Raw Potatoes)
- Geophagia (Earth, Soil, Or Clay)
- Hyalophagia (Glass)
- Lithophagia (Stones)
- Mucophagia (Mucus)
- Pagophagia (Ice)
- Plumbophagia (Lead)
- Trichophagia (Hair, Wool, And Other Fibers)
- Urophagia (Urine)
- Hematophagia (Vampirism) (Blood)

Diagnosis According to the DSM-5 criteria, for these behaviours to merit as pica, they must persist for more than one month. They have also to be appearing at an age when eating such objects is considered developmentally inappropriate (above 18 months of age) (Nasser et al., 2023) (King n.d)

Support for individuals with eating disorders

Individuals struggling with eating disorders usually benefit from treatments such as talking therapies, Cognitive Behavioural Therapy and Group therapies.

Substance Use Disorders.

These include alcohol use, opioids, stimulants, cannabis, and sedative use disorders
They take their names after the drug class involved. The symptoms presented also vary depending on the drug misused.

How does addiction come about? How do people get addicted to drugs/substances?

Substances that cause addiction are thought to cause structural changes in brain cells such that, the brain no longer responds the same way to the initial dose of medication that could have resulted in the desired response. As a result, the individual needs to take more of the drug to get the same desired effect. This is referred to as tolerance. At the same time, drugs of addiction tend to cause the body to release hormones that cause pleasurable feelings. When the drug wears off from the system, the individual feels horrible due to the absence of these hormones which had been produced in dysregulated abundance. This, together with the tolerance effect, result in the individual craving the drug for the need to have the pleasure. Ultimately this results in the need to take more of the drug to attain this desired feeling.

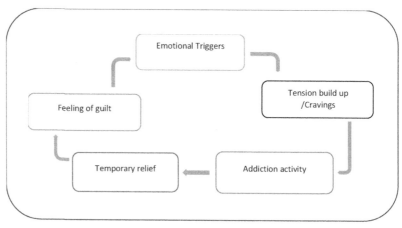

Figure 9 Diagram showing the addiction cycle

Addiction to substances does not happen with one time use. It takes a process that starts with contemplation, then experimenting one time. The person then begins to use the drug socially for recreation. If this is sustained, the person may begin to be a regular user, then enter the problem stage, where it is hard for them to go through the day without it. The next step thereafter is addiction.

Once addiction has been established in the psyche of an individual, it then follows a cycle of repetitive stages of an emotional trigger which causes a struggle within, creating tension to build up. Since most people use drugs as a stress coping mechanism, most will go ahead to use the drug for a quick fix to avoid dealing with the stressor. There will be a temporary relief from the tension and once the substance of abuse begins to wear off, the individual starts to have feelings of guilt. This, coupled with withdrawal symptoms can feed back into the cycle again as a trigger, then builds up the tension on and so on.

General signs of Addiction

Regardless of the drug being misused, the signs of addition are usually similar because of the shared cause and effect mechanism of addiction. Some of these may be noted by the individual themselves, friends, family or noted at workplace.

- Not remembering things that happen after drinking/using the drug
- Unable to stop using the drug despite knowing it is harming them
- Taking more than planned amount of the drug
- Feeling irritable when not high
- Frequent hangovers

- Giving up activities and work so you can go use the drug.
- Persistent cravings for drugs
- Needing more of the drug to get the same effect.
- Wanting to cut back but being unable to.

The DSM 5 classifies levels of addiction as shown below (Addiction Policy, 2022)

Categories of Symptoms

CATEGORIES OF SUD SYMPTOMS	Symptoms of substance use disorders in the DSM 5 fall into four categories: 1) impaired control; 2) social problems; 3) risky use, and 4) physical dependence.		
Impaired Control	Social Problems	Risky Use	Physical Dependence
Using more of a substance or more often than intended	Neglecting responsibilities and relationships	Using in risky settings	Needing more of the substance to get the same effect (tolerance)
Wanting to cut down or stop using but not being able to	Giving up activities they used to care about because of their substance use	Continued use despite known problems	Having withdrawal symptoms when a substance isn't used
	Inability to complete tasks at home, school or work		

Figure 10: Image curtesy of Addiction Policy Forum (2022)

Symptoms of Alcohol overdose (also seen in withdrawal)
- Anxiety.

- Depression.
- Irritability.
- Nausea, dry heaves.
- Racing heart.
- Restlessness.
- Shakiness.
- Sweating.
- Trouble sleeping.
- Seizures.
- Seeing things that are not there (hallucinations).
- Delirium tremens.
- Coma and death.

(Jung & Namkoong, 2014)

Symptoms of Opioid overdose (e.g. Morphine, tramadol, pethidine)

- Generally slowed down in movement and response to stimuli (sound, touch, or pain)
- Appears pale and feels clammy to touch.
- Blue/purple discoloration of fingernails or lips
- Nausea and vomiting
- Unable to be awaked or speak.
- Slowed down breathing (less than 12 breathes per minute)

(Bharat et al., 2021)

Symptoms of stimulant overdose (Cocaine, caffein, nicotine, methamphetamine)

- Hot, sweaty, or flashed skin
- Chest pain
- Unsteadiness
- Rigid muscles, tremors
- Or spasms
- Seizures
- Difficulty breathing

(Mansoor et al., 2022)

Symptoms of Cannabis use/overdose
- Hallucinations
- Fast heart rate
- Panic attacks
- Confusion
- Pale skin
- Headache

(Lake et al., 2020)

Symptoms of sedative overdose (Benzodiazepines e.g., diazepam, lorazepam)
- Slurred speech
- Ataxia (lack of coordination and balance)
- Slowed/ no response to stimuli(sound/touch/pain)

(CDC, 2021)

Diagnosis of drug abuse
- Urine and blood drug screens, Alco blow for alcohol.

What to do in overdose

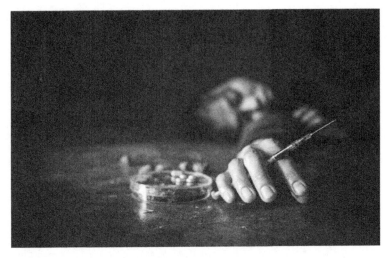

Figure 11: A drug user holding a syringe with needle and some pills on the floor: Image courtesy of Shutterstock

Drug overdose can be life threatening so act fast. If in the community or at home, Call for help on 111, 999, or any available emergency numbers. If in a hospital, inform the nurse in charge manager or doctors.

SOME ANTIDOTES USED IN MANAGEMENT OF DRUG OVERDOSE
- Benzodiazepines – Flumazenil

- Opioids – Naloxone

- Stimulants – Benzodiazepines

- Alcohol intoxication – Fomepizole

Support Available for Addition

Detox and rehabilitation services that may include psychological support and group therapies.
Recovery from addiction can be lengthy and cyclic. The person may have to go through several attempts before they succeed. See the image below for a brief illustration.

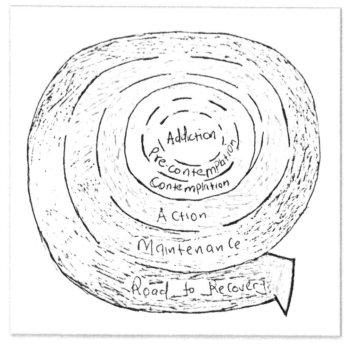

Figure 12 Showing the Addiction recovery spiral, sketch credits to D.I

Stages of addiction recovery

Just as it takes a while to get addicted to a substance, the recovery process equally is not instantaneous, at least not to most people. Usually, people struggle with episodes of success and relapse severally before they overcome it for a long time. When an individual gets to a point where they stay for six months without severe symptoms of dependence and or relapse into substance misuse, they are considered to be in recovery stage. But before they get here, they go through a few steps shown below proximate to the transtheoretical model of Prochaska and Velicer (1997) .

a) Addiction /precontemplation
This is when the individual is overly using the drug without thinking about the effects it has, there exists no desire to stop.

b) Contemplation
Here the person is thinking about stopping the habit. Sometimes it could come from medical advice, learning about effects of addiction, religious reasons or other reasons. The person is now looking into how to stop and where to get help.

c) Action
Now the addict is actively engaging in cessation programmes. This could be in a rehabilitation centre or by themselves in the comfort of their homes. This seems to work for people with milder forms of addiction. Severe symptoms benefit more in rehabilitation centers.

d) Maintenance/recovery
Here, the addict has done work on the problem and is now having a lot more days without the drug. There may be moment s of relapse, but great progress is being made towards the road to full recovery.

Axis 2: Personality Disorders, Autism Spectrum Disorders, Learning Disabilities And Mental Retardation

Personality Disorders

These are sets of deeply ingrained pattern of behaviour of certain nature that markedly deviates from what is considered acceptable behaviour/norms. These patterns appear to emerge during teenage and remain beyond this stage to adulthood and even old age. The patterns cause long-term difficulties in personal relationships and in general functioning of the individual in society'. These have been classified by the DSM 5 into 10 diagnoses. Below are the diagnoses outlined with their main features.

Paranoid

+ Believing that others are out to harm them or having hidden motives.
+ Hypersensitive to criticism
+ Becoming detached or socially isolated
+ Often argumentative and defensive
+ Having trouble relaxing

Support /therapies
+ Psychological support
+ Cognitive behavioural therapies

- Mindfulness therapies
- Relaxation techniques
- Medication

(Vyas & Khan, 2016) (Asensio-Aguerri et al., 2019)

Schizoid

- Lack of desire for close relationships
- Solitary
- Little or no interest in having sexual experiences
- Lacks close friends/confidants
- Indifferent to criticism or praise

Support /therapies
- Psychotherapy like talk therapy
- Group therapy
- Occupational support to learn social skills
- Medication

(Fariba et al., 2022)

Schizotypal

Has signs of schizoid Personality Disorder, accompanied with elements of paranoia, and hallucinations and/or delusions. May be seen as being on the same continuum with schizophrenia on the mild end of the spectrum.

Support /therapies
- Psychotherapy like CBT
- Occupational support to find work /skills that fit their personality
- Group therapy to learn social skills
- Medication

(Ettinger et al., 2014)

Antisocial

+ Ignoring or not awake to right and wrong
+ Lying often to take advantage of others
+ Disrespectful
+ Manipulative when they get chance
+ Being extremely opinionated
+ Problems with the law
+ Possible many crime records

Support /therapies

+ Psychotherapy like CBT
+ Schema therapy
+ Group therapy to learn social skills
+ Medication

(Black, 2015) (DeLisi et al., 2019)

Borderline /Emotionally Unstable Personality disorder (EUPD)

+ Emotional instability flipping through different emotions.
+ Disturbed patterns of thinking or perception (distortions) e.g., about self-image
+ Impulsive behaviour
+ Propensity for eating disorders
+ Intense but unstable relationships with others

Support /therapies

+ Dialectical Behavioural Therapy
+ Mentalization-Based Treatment
+ Transference-Focused Psychotherapy
+ Schema-Focused Therapy

- Medication

(Choi-Kain et al., 2017)

Histrionic

- Constantly seeking to be noticed e.g., extensive make up
- Seductive or sexually inappropriate behaviour
- Provocative behaviour
- Manipulative

Support /therapies

- CBT
- Psychodynamic psychotherapy to get at the root of emotions and behaviours
- Interpersonal therapy
- Medication for symptoms of depression

(Yurdagül et al., 2022) (Babl et al., 2022)

Narcissistic

- A strong sense of self-importance
- Exploits others for personal gain
- Preoccupation with power, beauty, or success
- Arrogant
- Lack empathy

Support /therapies

- Cognitive behavioural therapy
- Psychotherapy (talk)
- Gestalt therapy
- Schema therapy
- Transference-focused psychotherapy (TFP)
- Mentalization-based therapy (MBT)
- Dialectical behaviour therapy (DBT)

+ Metacognitive interpersonal therapy (MIT)
(Kiohan, 2023)

Avoidant

+ Low self-esteem
+ Prefers Self-isolation.
+ Avoiding interaction such as work, social, or school activities for fear of criticism or rejection

Support /therapies

+ Cognitive-behavioural therapy focused on social skills
+ Supportive psychotherapy
+ Psychodynamic psychotherapy
+ Anxiolytics and antidepressants

(Zimmerman, 2023)

Dependent

+ Marked difficulty in making decisions without help from others
+ Being either overly passive or submissive
+ Allowing or preferring other people to handle things on their behalf
+ Extreme fear of abandonment resulting in bad/exploitative relationships
+ Trouble carrying out tasks alone.
+ Avoids arguments preferring to agree rather than disagree with the opinions of other people

Support /therapies

+ Psychodynamic therapies
+ Cognitive behavioural therapy

+ Schema therapy
(Disney, 2013)

Obsessive compulsive personality disorder(OCPD)

+ Lack of flexibility
+ Overly devoted to work
+ Not being able to throw used/valueless things away
+ Not wanting to allow other people to do things for them
+ Not showing affection
+ Preoccupation with details, rules, and lists

Support /therapies
+ Cognitive Behavioural Therapy
+ Schema Therapy
(Gecaite-Stonciene et al., 2021)

Autism Spectrum Disorder

These are a group of disorders marked by repetitive patterns of behaviours of persistent difficulties with social communication and social interaction present since early childhood. They make it difficult for the individual to function normally on daily basis.

Other terms such as Asperger disorder', 'childhood disintegrative disorder' and 'Pervasive Developmental Disorder – Not Otherwise Specified (PDD-NOS) have been used before as a label denoting the level of difficulties encountered by the individual but DSM 5 seems to have collapsed these into one label 'autism spectrum disorder'

Features include

+ Anxious in social situations
+ Isolating self
+ Difficulty understanding the thoughts or feelings of other people
+ Difficulty in expressing how they feel
+ Difficulty understanding jokes such as sarcasm
+ Sticking to same routine, very anxious if it changes
+ Avoiding eye contact
+ Noticing details and patterns other people don't recognise

Symptoms see in childhood may include

+ Not responding to their name
+ Avoiding eye contact
+ Not smiling when smiled at
+ Getting very upset if they do not like a certain taste, smell or sound
+ Repetitive movements, such as flapping their hands, flicking their fingers or rocking their body
+ Not talking as much as other children

(NHS, 2022)

Support available for individuals with audism spectrum disorder

+ Behavioural management therapy
+ Cognitive behaviour therapy
+ Early intervention
+ Educational and school-based therapies

- Joint attention therapy
- Medication treatment to manage anxiety symptoms
- Nutritional therapy to broaden choice of food
- Occupational therapy to learn life skills

(NIH, 2021)

Learning Disabilities

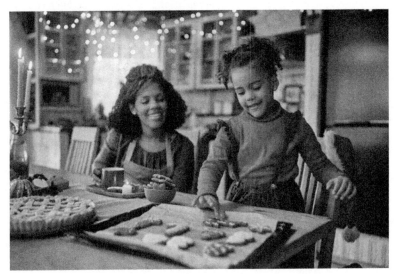

Figure 13 mother teaching her child cooking skills , photo credits to Shutterstock

These are conditions associated with reduced intellectual ability to learn new information or skills resulting in difficulty with everyday life since childhood. Some are discussed below

Learning Disability	Features
Dyslexia	• Problems spelling and writing • Difficulty reading • Mispronouncing names/words • Problems retrieving words during recall • Spending an unusually long-time completing tasks that involves reading or writing
Attention Deficit Hyperactivity Disorder (ADHD)	• Being restless with a short attention span • Constantly fidgeting • Impulsivity
Developmental Language Disorder (DLD)	• Disorganized storytelling • Limited use of complex sentences • Disorganised writing • Difficulty finding the right words • Difficulty with understanding figurative language • Reading problems • Frequent grammatical and spelling errors
Dysgraphia	• Difficulty with forming letters shapes • Awkward grip of writing tools e.g., pencils • Difficulty following a line or staying within margins • Trouble with sentence structure and rules of grammar.

Others include:

Developmental Coordination Disorder (DCD)- difficulty with movement and co-ordination affecting performance of activities of daily living
Dyscalculia- this is difficulty specific to numbers and mathematical problems.

Mental Retardation/Intellectual Disabilities

This is below average intellectual ability that occurs alongside deficits in at least two or more of the following skills: communication, social skills, self-care, self-direction, living skills, health and safety, academic, work and leisure. There are a number of diagnosable conditions associated with mental retardation/intellectual disabilities. These include Fragile X syndrome, Down Syndrome, Neurofibromatosis, Congenital hypothyroidism, Foetal alcohol spectrum disorder, Williams syndrome, Phenylketonuria (PKU), Prader-Willi Syndrome.

What support is available for learning disabilities and mental retardation?

For all the learning disabilities, support will focus on tailoring living and learning methods according to the individual's leaning needs. An individual with mild difficulties may only require a little support while those with severe needs will require a more complex plan. This could be a collaboration between learning institutions, therapists, community teams and parents/care givers.

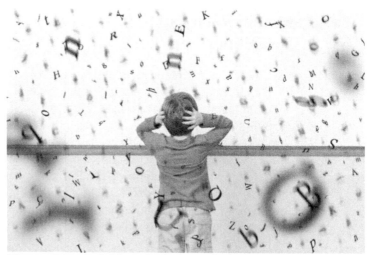

Figure 14: A child with dyslexia before a whiteboard unable to read flying letters; image courtesy of Shutterstock

Non-Suicidal Self-Injury Disorder (formerly self-harm)

This is a condition characterised with the urge to harm one's own body without the intent of killing self. This may be accomplished through physical injury such as cutting, head banging or non-lethal ingestion of drugs. The condition appears to occur more among adolescents than the other age groups.

Diagnosis

The behaviour has to occur at least 5 separate days in the last 12 months. The behaviour should also be accompanied by frequent thoughts of harming self with or without them being acted upon. The behaviour also needs to be affecting academics or other areas of functioning and be done when seeking to obtain some kind of relief from when faced with a difficulty, or to induce a positive feeling. Also, it has to not be better explained by any other mental health issue as fitting the criterion for the other illness, such as obsessions/compulsions or other issues like hair pulling.

Support available for non-suicidal self Injury
- Psychotherapy to find the route course of the problem
- Inpatient care to help manage symptoms
- Medication to manage other underlying mental illnesses

(Brager-Larsen et al., 2023) (Zetterqvist et al., 2020) (MayoClinic, 2023)

Suicide Behaviour Disorder (SBD)

Suicidal behaviour disorder is a spectrum of behaviours ranging from suicide ideation, suicide attempt and preparatory behaviours all the way to completed suicide. Suicidal ideation refers to the process of thinking, considering, or planning a suicide. Suicidal takes over a million lives worldwide yearly while non-fatal suicidal behaviour is estimated to be 50 times more common and is probably underreported.

Individuals with substance abuse, Bipolar mood disorder with psychotic features, psychotic disorders and major depressive disorders are at the highest risk of suicide ideation and attempts.

Early warning signs for possible suicide ideation
- Talking about wanting to die
- Displaying feelings of guilt, shame or being a burden to others
- Hopelessness, feeling trapped, or having no reason to live
- Emotionally feeling extremely sad, anxious, agitated, or full of rage
- Unbearable physical pain
- Planning or researching ways to die
- Withdrawing from friends, saying goodbye, giving away important items, or making a will
- Taking dangerous risks such as driving extremely fast
- Using drugs or alcohol more often

(Baldessarini & Tondo, 2020) (Moutier, 2023) (NIH, n.d)

Support Available for Suicide Behaviour Disorder
- If a person you know displays any of these symptoms highlighted and you are concerned about them, please ring emergency services for help. If in the hospital, please inform clinical staff on shift.
- Psychotherapy is available for mild forms of ideation
- Medication to manage symptoms of underlying illnesses
- Inpatient support to eliminate available options for suicide attempt

CAUSES OF MENTAL HEALTH PROBLEMS

There is no definite single cause of mental health problems. It is theorised that a combination of factors works together in someway to result in mental illness. An individual who has lived their lives relatively stable till adulthood may suddenly begin to exhibit signs of mental illness. In such a case, it becomes difficult to conclude the cause of this onset. Any of the theorised explanations could fit; it could be biological predisposition, social, or stemming from psychological wellbeing.

Biological causes are developmental/structural problems that may have been passed on to the individual from parent to offspring through genetic composition. They could also be other issues that resulted in altered development, e.g., illness of mother during pregnancy impacting on child development. **Social factors** may include interactions such as poor living conditions or peer influence in use of drugs of abuse. **Psychological** may be loss of a loved one, childhood trauma or any major event that affects psychological stability.

Because of the hardship of finding the accurate cause of mental illness, clinicians have come up with a conceptual framework that helps understand the patient. They look at the person with these broad topics in mind;

Predisposing factors – features that place the person at risk of developing illness (the social, biological, psychological)

Precipitating factors -Usually events that took place shortly before onset of illness; usually a major stressor or drug overdose

Perpetuating factors – Things that feed into/maintain the existence of the illness once it has begun e.g., unaddressed conflicts, financial deprivation, etc

Protective factors- these help the individual cope with the illness and potentially push them towards recovery. For example, learning stress coping skills, exercise and community support

How do patients end up in mental health services?

There are two main ways a person may become a service user. This is defined by the law of the land for example the Mental health act of 1983 for the United Kingdom.

a) **Voluntary treatment** where the individual realises that they need support and they approach mental health services for help. They may be admitted in hospital for a period then discharged at their own request.

b) The other option **is involuntary treatment** where an individual who may be a risk to themselves or others is taken into services by the police, relatives, well-wishers or the crisis response team. The individual will be detained for a given period until they get better before they are discharged back to the community or referred to specialised services.

In practice, a voluntary patient walks in on their own accord and could leave at their own free will, while an involuntary patient is detained against their own will (put under a section of mental health law). In these circumstances their rights are being restricted thus there is need for more than one doctor to assess the patient. If both doctors agree that the individual needs to be detained, they will set the duration of time they require. For example, a maximum of 28 days for assessment, then 6 months for treatment. If the patient won't have recovered enough to go back to the community, the psychiatrist could extend this period for another 6 months. It is worthwhile to check and confirm this from the mental health law of your country to see the accurate prescriptions in that law.

DIFFERENT UNITS OFFERING CARE

For ease of explanation, I will use the United Kingdom setup to explain this part.

Accident and emergency departments (A&E)

These are not mental heath units; however, they receive all manner of patients. Sometimes relatives could walk in with a restrained patient seeking help, or a voluntary patient could also come in to seek help. Here, they might get emergency services then be referred to the best available option for them such as *acute wards*

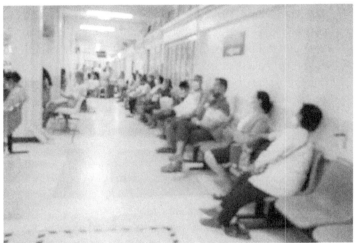

Figure 15: Image of patients waiting to be seen in an emergency department: image courtesy of Shutterstock

Acute wards

These accommodate both voluntary and involuntary patients. The main aim here is to are provide a stabilising environment that is safe for persons in a mental crisis. You may look at it as a unit handling mental health emergencies. If a patient in this setting is considered to require more support, they may be moved up one level to *Psychiatric Intensive Care Units (PICU)*

PICU (Psychiatric Intensive Care Units)

These units are modelled to provide more intensive assessment and comprehensive treatment to individuals with serious mental health issues. They have more restrictions including movement, utilisation of items like blades and glasses.

This helps individuals to stabilise but still be able to access what they need for personal care and comfort. Is not unusual to see many patients here managed on enhanced levels of observation such as eyesight/constant engagements or in more secure parts of the ward called seclusion suits. Indeed, all mental health units have these suits. We will see what they are later in the book.

Specialist wards

Some individuals have a set of symptoms or features that are rather peculiar and being in general mental health units will often not offer the best support for them. Such individuals are supported in specialised mental health units. Examples of such wards would be Child and Adolescent Mental Health Services (CAHMS), eating disorder, learning disability and personality disorder wards. Here, specialists will have training specific to meet their need. Policies here will also often be drafted in a manner to create the most appropriate environments to support them.

Rehabilitation centres

These are units specialised in supporting people with addictions to minimise or cease using drugs/object of addiction. They have programmes such as extensive detox that may be particularly difficult for people to do successfully by themselves in the community. Here, they get to meet peers doing the same treatments and this somewhat provides group therapy support which enhances compliance.

Prisons

This is also not a mental health unit. However, many individuals who are arrested for crime may be subjected to mental health assessments. Some turn out to have mental health illnesses. Some studies have shown that more than a quarter of prisoners have some sort of mental health problem that could be correlated to their crimes. This then makes it worthwhile to consider this as an important part of mental health institutions that one would work in.

Care /Nursing homes

This is also not particularly a mental health unit, but it has residents who may or may not be affected by some aspects that relate to the mental health act. Individuals in a care home are usually people who need some form of support to live and function including accommodation, personal care, and medication. A large number may be senior citizens suffering from conditions such as dementia and may sometimes lack the capacity to make decisions about their own care. As a result, they are covered by a law called Mental capacity act, which relates to the Mental Health Act because the individuals as at that moment have been deprived of their liberty to make decisions about their own lives. Extensive training is done for staff about this before they start working so just ask about it if no one has mentioned it to you if you yet.

MEDICATION USED IN MANAGEMENT OF MENTAL HEALTH CONDITIONS

Antidepressants

There are 5 classes of these medications. Each class works in a different way to increase the availability of neurotransmitters implicated in depression.

a) Selective Serotonin Reuptake Inhibitors (SSRIs) – prevent reuptake of serotonin making it more readily available for use. Examples Are Citalopram, Escitalopram, Fluvoxamine, Paroxetine, Fluoxetine, Vilazodone and Sertraline

b) Serotonin and Norepinephrine Reuptake Inhibitors (SNRIs)- work as SSRIs but also prevent reuptake of norepinephrine. Examples are duloxetine, venlafaxine, levomilnacipran, desvenlafaxine, and milnacipran

c) Tricyclic Antidepressants (TCAs)- Acts like SNRIs but also prevents reuptake of acetylcholine. Examples are clomipramine, amoxapine, amitriptyline, desipramine, nortriptyline, doxepin, trimipramine, imipramine, protriptyline

d) Monoamine Oxidase Inhibitors (MAOIs)- Blocks the action of monoamine oxidase enzyme that breaks down monoamines (dopamine, serotonin, norepinephrine), thus they remain bioavailable for longer.

e) Atypical antidepressants – Have varied ways of managing depression symptoms. Trazodone and vortixetine prevents reuptake of serotonin and blocks adrenaline receptors, Mirtazapine blocks adrenergic brain receptors and bupropion prevents reuptake of dopamine (Schimelpfening, 2022)

Common side effects of antidepressants to look out for

Each class of antidepressants will have a certain variation of side effects. Here are some common ones that may be shared by most of them.

+ Increased risk for type two diabetes
+ Decreased alertness, thus need to avoid driving especially when taking them for the first time
+ Increased risk for Gastrointestinal bleeds
+ Hypomania – A high level of energy that affects ability to concentrate or carry out daily activities

- Neuroleptic malignant syndrome - is characterised by sweating, tremor, rapid heartbeat, confusion, stiffness/rigidity. This is a medical emergency that should involve stopping the assaulting drug, and supportive measures such as rehydration and cooling of the body to reduce damage to tissues. Bromocriptine and dantoline may be used to manage severe symptoms. (Berman, 2011)
- Serotonin syndrome - this is another life-threatening side effect. It has similar signs with NMS like tremor, sweating, rapid heartbeat and confusion. However, this includes involuntary muscle twitches, convulsions, arrythmias, or coma. This is another medical emergency.

Antipsychotics /neuroleptics

There are two classes, both named by the period in which they were discovered. First generation (typical) were the first to be developed, and second generation (Atypical) came later on. The main difference between the two however comes in the lower propensity of the second-generation neuroleptics in causing tardive dyskinesia (Ameer & Saadabadi, 2023).

Examples of these medication include.

Typical neuroleptics - Chlorpromazine, Droperidol, Fluphenazine, Haloperidol, Loxapine, Perphenazine, Pimozide, Prochlorperazine, Thioridazine, Thiothixene, Trifluoperazine

Atypical neuroleptics – Aripiprazole, Clozapine, Quetiapine, Olanzapine, Cariprazine, Asenapine, Risperidone, Lumateperone, Paliperidone, Pimavanserin, Iloperidone

Common side effects of antipsychotics
- dizziness
- weight gain
- blurred vision
- movement effects (for example, tremor, stiffness, agitation)
- sedation (low energy and sleepiness)
- loss of menstrual periods in women
- fluid retention
- dry mouth
- sexual dysfunctions
- headaches

(Stroup & Gray, 2018)

Anxiolytics

Different classes of medication can be used in management of anxiety disorders . Anxiolytics(benzodiazepines), beta blockers , Antidepressants and buspirone

a) Anxiolytics – Also called sedatives, work by enhancing the binding of an inhibitory neurotransmitter in the brain called Gamma Aminobutyric Acid (GABA), thus slowing down brain activity. Because of this mechanism of action, these drugs tend to make one sleepy and if taken in large quantities could slow or completely shut down vital functions like breathing (Gancher, 2010). Examples include, Diazepam, Chlordiazepoxide, Clonazepam, Quazepam, Oxazepam, Lorazepam and Alprazolam

b) Beta blockers – Propranolol and Atenolol are prescribed off label to manage anxiety symptoms. They act by preventing the binding of catecholamines (like adrenaline) to receptors that would effect symptoms of anxiety such as increased hear and breathing rate and breakdown of glucose to make it available for fight /flight.

c) Antidepressants – these take a minimum of 4 weeks to have noticeable results, but are suitable for long term use unlike benzodiazepines and beta blockers which may be effective to manage acute symptoms but may not be perfect for prolonged daily use. SNRIs (for Generalised anxiety disorders), Tricyclics (for OCD), MOIs for phobias and panic attacks

d) Buspirone – this is an anxiolytic but has a different mechanism of action to benzodiazepines, thus classed separately. It suppresses serotonergic activity and increases dopaminergic and noradrenergic activities in the brain (Eison & Temple, 1986).

Common side effects
+ Slurred speech.

- Low heart rate.
- Low blood pressure.
- Irregular breathing.
- Memory loss.
- Confusion.
- Depression.
- Dizziness.

(Whitten, 2023)

Mood Stabilizers

These are medications used in management of bipolar mood disorder, mania, hypomania, severe depression and schizoaffective disorder. They are derived from different classes of drugs because of their ability to also help in mood dysregulation disorders. Examples are Lithium, Anti-convulsant (carbamezipine, lamotrigine, sodium valproate), Antipsychotics (haloperidol, olanzapine, quetiapine, and risperidone (Mind, 2020).

Overall, their mechanism of action revolves around minimising excitatory activities of glutamate neurotransmitter in the brain, and enhancing activity of GABA usually in a way to strike a balance which is achieved by the clinician titrating the dosage to the point where it is deemed to be most effective with minimal side effects.

Common side effects
- Weight gain
- GI disturbances
- Hepatotoxicity and Renal toxicity

(Nath & Gupta, 2023)

Stimulants

Three types of stimulants, amphetamine (dextro-amphetamine and levo-amphetamine), Methamphetamine and methylphenidate (dextro-methylphenidate and levo-methylphenidate), may be used for treatment of attention deficit/hyperactivity disorder (ADHD), management of narcolepsy (sleep disorder) or weight reduction in obesity. These drugs work by increasing amount of catecholamines in the brain which helps in ADHD by increasing levels of attention, increasing availability of dopamine in the brain thus enhancing alertness/wakefulness, and increasing energy expenditure while reducing food intake, and in (Archer et al., 2016) (Brown et al., 2017)

Common side effects

- Decreased appetite
- Anxiety.
- Jitteriness.
- Headaches.
- Weight loss.
- Insomnia.
- Psychosis.
- Pruritus

(Farzam et al., 2023)

Medication used in management of seizures.

They are also called anticonvulsant medication. Three main classes exist based on their mode of action.

Effect on ion channels [essentially blocks the ion channels reducing their activity]	Effect of Gamma aminobutyric acid (GABA) [Enhances binding of this inhibitory neurotransmitter]	Effects on excitatory amino acids (glutamate and aspartate) [reduces activity of these excitatory neurotransmitters]
Na⁺ • Phenytoin • Carbamazepine • Lamotrigine • Valproic acid Ca⁺ • Ethosuximide • valproic acid	• **Benzodiazepines** (lorazepam, diazepam midazolam) • Barbiturates (phenobarbitone) • Gabapentin • Vigabatrin	• Topiramate • Felbamate (Tadvi, 2016) (Davies, 1995)

Common side effects of anticonvulsants
+ Nausea
+ abdominal pain
+ dizziness
+ sleepiness
+ irritability
+ anxiety
+ mood changes

(RCH), (Mutanana et al., 2020)

Medication used in management of Parkinson's disease

Because the primary reason for symptoms is lack of dopamine in parts of the brain stem, medication used in managing the symptoms of Parkinson's disease and parkinsonism work by increasing the availability of dopamine by acting as agonists, or inhibiting degradation of available dopamine such as inhibiting the activities of Monoamine oxidase enzyme. Examples of medication include

a) Dopamine precursor- Levodopa
b) Dopamine agonists – Ropinirole, Bromocriptine, Pramipexole
c) MAO B inhibitors – Selegiline
d) Dopamine facilitator – Amantadine
e) Peripheral decarboxylase inhibitors- Carbidopa, Benserazide
f) COMT inhibitors – Entacapone, Tolcapone

Common side effects
+ Dizziness
+ Orthostatic hypertension
+ Insomnia
+ Blurry vision
+ Hypersexuality
(APDA, 2023)

Drugs used in management of Alzheimer's

The drugs used to manage Alzheimer's are classified in two ways based on their mechanism of action. These are Acetylcholinesterase inhibitors/cholinesterase inhibitors and NMDA receptor antagonists. The medications are meant to address the two main issues in this disease which are:
  a) Lack of acetylcholine
  b) Excessive production of glutamate to compensate for lack of acetylcholine, but excess amount of it damages more nerves that use acetylcholine

Cholinesterase inhibitors (like donepezil, rivastigmine, galantamine) prevent the breakdown acetylcholine thus causing it to be available in the brain for use.

N-methyl-D-aspartate (NMDA) receptor antagonists (Memantine) prevent the binding of glutamate to the glutamate receptor thus prevents its excessive action in Alzheimer. (Alzheimers.org, 2014)

Common side effects
  - Dizziness
  - Headache
  - Confusion
  - Agitation

(Mayoclinic, 2023)

Anticholinergics

These are a class of medication used only to manage episodes of extrapyramidal side effects and should not be used routinely due to their associated effects of worsening symptoms of psychotic disorders (WHO, 2012). Their mechanism of action is by reducing cholinergic activity which includes skeletal muscle contraction that is excessive in EP (Jett, 1998). Procyclidine, benztropine and trihexyphenidyl are the most utilised medication for this purpose.

Common side effects of anticholinergics
- Dry Mouth
- Constipation
- Urinary Retention
- Bowel Obstruction
- Dilated Pupils
- Blurred Vision
- Increased Heart Rate
- Decreased Sweating

(Lieberman, 2004)

OTHER THERAPY OPTIONS AVAILABLE MANAGEMENT OF MENTAL HEALTH CONDITIONS

Psychotherapy

This form of therapy involves talking to clients by establishing a therapeutic relation where they can be able to share thoughts and feelings with the therapist in confidence. It is also known as talk therapy or psychological counselling. The aims of treatment include;

+ Creating trusting relationships beginning with one with the therapist
+ Identify and manage underlying issues that trigger self-injury, anxiety or other distress
+ Learning coping skills to better manage distress
+ Learning how to boost your self-image and self esteem

- Developing skills to improve social skills.
- Developing healthy problem-solving skills.

There a number of psychotherapies , some are listed below.

i. Cognitive Behavioural Therapy (CBT)- whose main focus is to identify unhealthy, negative beliefs and behaviours and replace them with more effective ones.

ii. Dialectical Behaviour Therapy, a type of CBT that teaches behavioural skills to help you handle distress, manager or regulate your emotions, and improve your relationships with others.

iii. Mindfulness-Based Therapies, that help in learning how to be aware of self and to reduce automatic impulsive responses.

iv. Schema Therapy – these are talk therapies that focus on beliefs and structures that individuals have developed in themselves over the years since childhood. These schemas are the ones that the individual uses to view the world thus forming a self-concept which informs their thought processes and behaviours.

Relaxation therapy

These are a group of therapies that focus on reducing the body's stress response by lowering the respiration rate, heart rate and blood pressure. This opposes the stress response initiated by the body like in anxiety and panic disorders. Examples include Progressive Relaxation, Autogenic Training, Guided Imagery, Biofeedback-Assisted Relaxation, Self-Hypnosis, yoga and Breathing Exercises.

Eye Movement Desensitization and Reprocessing (EMDR)

This is a type of relaxation therapy that is more specifically used in PTSD. The therapist offers different techniques to the patient that involves moving they eyes with eyes closed to release tension in muscles and to retrain the body into overcoming flashbacks, nightmares, and disturbing images.

Aromatherapy, music therapy and massage

Aromatherapy involves the use of essential oils and scents to improve physical, emotional, and spiritual wellbeing. Music therapy is the use of music in form of composing, listening, or improvising on music with the help of a music therapist. Massage therapy involves rubbing and kneading muscles of the body to relive tension that builds up in stressful situations. All of these therapies use the same principle of causing the body to produce hormones (like endorphins) that cause relaxation and comfort thus countering distress and anxiety.

Exposure therapy

this is a type of therapy where the individual is exposed to the things and situations they fear. The aim is to create a trusting safe environment in which these exposures are done with the hope of decreasing the amount of anxiety to build resilience in phobias, post-traumatic stress disorder (PTSD) and panic disorders.

(NIH, n.d) (WebMD, 2023) (NCBI, n.d) (Montgomery, 2016) (Shacknai, 2020) (APA, 2017)

ROLES OF SERVICE PROVIDERS

There are a ton of professionals who work with every individual patient. Each professional and worker knows their roles. Some roles may appear to be shared, and this sometimes causes minor conflicts at work. However, it does not have to be this way. It should, on the contrary, help in merging efforts of care providers to improve on efficiency.

We will now briefly look at the different groups of people working in these services and their roles. You will soon see that because of this division of labour, it might not be as hard as it may appear. Nurses, doctors, consultants, support workers, psychologists, occupational therapy, case managers, activity co-ordinators, advocacy, pharmacy, dieticians, podiatrists, are some of the common cadres you will encounter on the regular.

Nurses

These are probably the largest group of qualified professionals working in most health care settings. This means their practice is closely monitored by a nursing regulatory body in the states they work in. This happens after they have undergone training in colleges or universities, and thereafter get registered and are issued with a license/pin number. The purpose is to ensure every practitioner practices safely, does their best not to harm patients, and acts to benefits those under their care. If gross misconduct is reported, an investigation is initiated against the professional. Where evidence is found to support the allegations, they are struck off from the register ad can no longer practice as qualified professionals.

There is a code of practice that helps to demarcate functions. Doctors, pharmacists, occupational therapists, dieticians, psychologists and many other trained professionals are also registered by their own professional bodies. In the UK, nurses are registered with the Nursing and Midwifery council (NMC), in the USA, each state has its own Board of Nursing, Australia has its Nursing and Midwifery Board of Australia, Nursing Council of Hong Kong in China, and Nursing and Midwifery Council of Nigeria. Overall, it will bear the name of the country or state somewhere in it.

Different jurisdictions have their own prescribed roles for nurses; however, these are what would be considered general responsibilities that nurses are expected to carry out in mental health units.

+ Administer medication.
+ Consult /coordinate with other health care professionals
+ Educate patients and staff

- Planning/ be in charge of shifts and supervise personnel on the shift
- Be the primary/immediate patient advocate.
- Develop care plans
- Monitor progress of patients e.g., vital signs
- Maintaining patient records
- Taking the leadership role in emergencies such as fire, first aid, chocking etc
- Have holding powers for mentally ill patients who are a risk to self and others.
- Leading roles in care co-ordination and multidisciplinary meetings.

Doctors And Consultants

Just like nurses, these too are registered professionals. Examples of bodies that register them include the National Medical Commission in India (NMC), the Brazilian Federal Council of Medicine (BFCM), the Medical Board of California (MBC) and the General Medical Council (GMC) in the UK

The roles of doctors include
- Assess patients of various ailments and symptoms
- Prescribe care and medication
- Order and review tests
- Consult with other clinicians and professionals
- Review patients to track progress

Consultants are doctors who have gained more training in specific areas of medicine. They are often referred to depending on their area of specialization. In mental health, you may encounter forensic psychiatrists, childhood and adolescent psychiatrist, learning disabilities psychiatrist and many more. Psychiatrists are rally the main prescribers of care in mental health. They carry out mental health assessments and may offer a diagnosis for a cluster of behaviours. The rest of the health care team then works with this diagnosis to finds the best approach to support the service user.

Support Worker, Nursing Assistant, Nursing Auxiliary, Health Care Assistants

This role is not for registered staff. However, it forms the backbone of all care in the services. Support workers are involved in almost everything. You will see them working with the other professionals, most of the time carrying out supervised tasks. In general, their daily roles include but not limited to;

- Maintaining clean working environments
- Monitoring and doing basic health checks
- Making patients feel comfortable.
- Helping patients who cannot move to ambulate or exercise
- Washing and dressing patients
- Serving meals
- Helping to feed patients who cannot do it themselves
- Escorting patients on leave
- Helping with all other activities of daily living (ADLs)

Psychology

These are registered professionals who also engage with patients to offer psychological therapy and counselling services. Their roles may include

+ Assessing patients with psychological problems
+ Prescribing and offering psychological treatments
+ Teaching and training staff
+ Supporting staff during debriefs, supervision, or when struggling
+ May be involved in research and other studies in the healthcare setting

Pharmacists

These are individuals whose roles are tailored towards medication and substances used in treatments. Their roles are to:

+ Dispense prescribed medication
+ check quality of medicines supplied
+ Ensure safety of medicines prescribed to patients
+ Educate staff and patients about medication safety, side effects, storage, etc
+ Ensure all prescriptions are within the law

Occupational Therapists

The main role of these professionals is to support patients to adapt to new lives that are due to emerging difficulties . This could include for example helping a person who is recovering from a stroke to adapt to their home or vehicle to make them more accessible. Other roles include;

+ Helping people with disability to adjust with their difficulty
+ Prescribing specialist equipment such as those needed for mobility, sleep or work
+ Helping people to cope with memory or sensory loss
+ Helping people learn living skills like cooking, budgeting, washing etc

Speech and Language Therapists

They provide assessment, treatment and support for people with difficulties with speech, eating, drinking and swallowing. They may engage in treatments such as

+ Breathing exercises
+ Swallowing
+ Voice training
+ Facial massage

Case Managers

These are individuals who may be clinical professionals such as nurses, psychologists or any other university-trained persons in a healthcare related field whose main role is to oversee that the patient is getting the best care they deserve. They may be concerned with every detail of care and are particularly keen to make sure client needs are not neglected and that the team is doing their best to support them. Roles include to:

- Assess client treatment needs
- Create and evaluate care plans
- Leasing and advocating between clinicians and patients
- Monitor rehabilitation programmes
- Review documents and records

We also have other professionals such as dieticians, podiatrist, advocacy, activity co-ordinators and others. Their roles tend to reflect in their titles and thus you might find it easier to understand the role they play the more you work together with them.

PATIENT SITUATIONSHIPS TO BE AWARE OF

Sometimes unexpected occurrences happen when working with patients. If you are unprepared, you may be caught off guard not knowing what to do. Here are some of them.

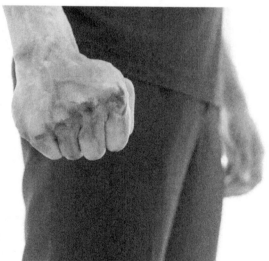

Figure 16: A man with blood on his knuckles after assaulting someone, example of when not to engage: Image curtesy of Shutterstock

The violent patient/aggressive/abusive patient

Some patients because of their severity of illness may come across as aggressive or even violent. It is of great interest that staff approach aggressive patients with caution, and with de-escalation skills commensurate to the situation. It is important that you do not do this alone. Get colleagues to be with you if you are the one having to engage with the patient. This makes sure that if events escalate undesirably, you will have people to protect you from aggression and eliminate the possibility of false accusation from service users who may interpret your interaction differently due to illness, malice or dislike for whatever reason.

There is training offered in de-escalation that should equip you with the tools you need to handle such situations. The bottom line is, you will never be alone, and you should never be alone with an aggressive patient (or any patient) in isolated places where help is out of reach. If you realise you are alone, back off in a calm manner and call for help.

If the service user is aggressive/violent and has a weapon with them, do not engage. Monitor the situation to ensure they are not harming themselves or others and call the police.

The dead patient

As unfortunate as it may be, some of the service users either due to old age, chronic disease, prognosis, drug abuse or self-harm/suicidal behaviour; some end up dying.

For this explanation, we will work with the assumption that you are first on sight. At the exact moment you first see the service user in a state that you suspect death/loss of consciousness, the fact remains that you are not sure if they are alive, neither are you sure that they are dead.

- The first thing you need to do is call/shout/buzz for help.
- At the same time assess the area quickly for any possible sources of danger such as naked electrical wires, sharp tools, blood/body fluids etc. Always remember that your safety is the most important thing at that time.
- Remember the units have other service users too who may be curious to know why you are calling for help. Try as much as possible to control human traffic to keep service users away from the scene.
- Manage the patient/body together as a team. Offer CPR if they do not have a DNR, and proceed with procedures as per our policies
- If the patient is confirmed dead make sure to leave the room/area as locked if that is possible or protected from the public until the police arrive to check the area.
- Remember to leave only with the equipment you came in with, DO NOT clean the room or rearrange it since the state of the room/scene is part of evidence.

The patient that runs away/ escapes

Sometimes service users find opportunities to run away. It could be from the unit, or during escorted leave outside the unit.

If the service user is able to converse with you, try to remind them of the consequences of their action. If they still run off, do not chase after them because doing so endangers both their safety and your own safety like on the road with all the traffic. Only contact the unit, inform the charge nurse/most senior staff on the shift, and ring the police to inform them about the incident. Remember to record the time and location of last interaction.

Escalation and de-escalation of frustrated/angry service users

Escalation

+ These are all the things you are not supposed to do when attempting to defuse a situation where a person is angry, agitated, or frustrated.
+ Being in a threatening body language such as facial expressions ad or raising your voice
+ Challenge the patient/angry person
+ Respond to a threat with a threat
+ Invalidate or demean their concerns
+ Interrupting when they are talking intentionally/repetitively

+ Turning /giving them your back/not in your visual field

De-escalation

The above actions will only make the patient see you as picking sides with the person /situation that they are angry at and thus class you together with it. You might just be added on the list of things they want to knock out. Instead, you need to enter the scene with this skillset, knowing that the reason the person is aggressive is possibly them being in distress over something, or experiencing some form of fear and frustration. Empathy and effective communication cannot be underestimated for these kind of scenarios.

+ Stay calm
+ Listen to what the issue is – do not assume you are aware of what happened, even if you have received a report from someone else.
+ Maintain a safe distance, not too close in their personal space, be atleat one and hald meters/5 feet away. This helps to make them feel safe, and also gives you time to react if they launch towards you.
+ maintain appropriate eye contact to connect with the person
+ use active listening skills like leaning forward to show you are attentive. Repeat/rephrase what they have told you to make sure you get it clearly, nod to show you are getting wat they are saying.
+ Express empathy commensurate to the situation

- Validate their feelings with words like ' I understand why you felt so angry after....' 'I see why you felt that way...' , ' that must have been very difficult for you...'
- When asking questions, use short sentences, and be clear with tone and volume because if they cant hear you it might add onto the list of frustrations
- Remember that the person is angry at the moment, and its hard for them to reason with logic, so don't push logic into the argument, offer short term solutions that can resolve the immediate problem, then create time later to discuss logic when the situation has long been diffused.

THE WORK ENVIRONMENT

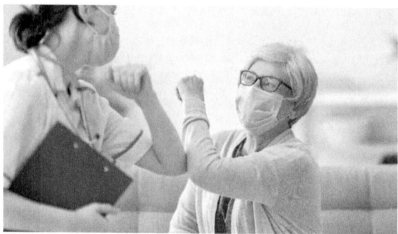

Figure 17: Staff and patient using elbows to greet each other to avoid handshake: Image courtesy of Shutterstock

Infection Control

Infections are a big thing in hospitals. One service user with a contagious disease could very easily pass it on to peers and even staff because of how close people work together in sharing equipment and shared spaces.

If more patients get the same infection, then this only strains the existing physical and human resources. Also, as collateral, if staff also get ill and have to ring in sick or altogether cancel shifts due to fear of contacting a disease, this only makes things worse. As a consequence, strict infection prevention guidelines are put in place by your employer to minimise the risk of cross infections in workplaces.

Patients may require quarantine or self-isolation in bedspaces sometimes, and staff let go off the shift if they exhibit signs of contagious diseases such as Covid 19 or diarrhoea. Waste segregation, surface cleaning schedules and so on should be clearly made aware to all staff to minimise these risks. Be sure to know the policies regarding this in your workplace.

General Principles of Infection Prevention and Control

Understanding the infection chain is a helpful aid to critical thinking among staff. Below is a diagram showing the relationship between the elements involved in the chain.

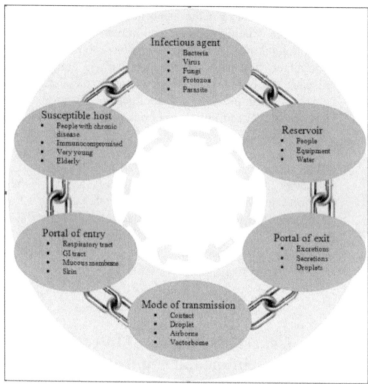

Figure 18: Credits to the Northern Ireland Region Infection Prevention and Control Manual

Having seen the infection cycle, it is key to understand how to disrupt the chain effectively. We achieve this by;

+ The infectious agent is eliminated - by treating infected people, water sources or surfaces where they may be reserved.
+ The portal of exit is managed through good infection prevention and control practices (e.g., hand hygiene, appropriate use of PPE, safe packaging and disposal of waste)

- Protecting the portal of entry (e.g., Aseptic non-touch technique, safe catheter care, wound care)
- Reducing the susceptibility of patients receiving healthcare (e.g., treatment of underlying disease, recognising high risk patients, proper nutrition and exercise)

Documentation

In general, anything not documented is considered not done. Lack of documentation appear as if you did nothing on your shift. Just remember documentation is part of the job. Make sure you've documented and signed all things you need to document.

These are two special documents you need to be aware off as they contain specific information about the patient: DNACPR and advanced statements.

a) **DNACPR** or just DNR is Do not attempt cardiopulmonary resuscitation. If a client has this in place, If they are seen to appear to be dying, the staff are prohibited from attempting to offer CPR. Most of these will be individuals advanced in age or with a long-standing chronic illness.

b) **Advanced statement** – this is a document listing wishes of the client about future care when they might not have the capacity to make their own statements. This might contain information about who may make decisions for the client at such times. It could be a 'next of kin', 'nearest relative' or any nominated individual by the service user.

Seclusions and Long-term segregation suites

These are special rooms set apart to support those who are struggling more than others on the unit and particularly present as being a risk to themselves or others if they remain on the normal ward environment. A decision to send one to seclusion will be made by the nurses or the doctors. If it was decided by the nurse, a doctor has to review the patient within an hour and reviewed by a consultant within 24 hours. Placement in seclusion may be for a brief moment and ends as soon as the presentation of the patient changes and the level of risk that caused them to be sent into it has changed. On other occasions, a patient may stay for prolonged periods like months and years. The clinical team in these occasions may decide to support the client in lesser restrictive environments called long term segregation. This is any setting that is generally more comfortable than seclusion suit that only has a mattress and toilet behind a locked door. For LTS, the patient may have a few rooms top themselves such as lounge, secure garden to get some fresh air, and a bedspace.

In both scenarios, the patient is assessed as not ready to go back on the ward as they still have risks towards self or others. Staff should always keep the service user in their eyesight, whether they are awake or asleep. It helps that sometimes CCTVs are available to offer more views of the patient whilst in seclusion.

Safeguarding Issues

Service users under our care depend on us for safety alongside therapy and other services we offer. It is sad to say that sometimes due to short staffing or irresponsibility on the part of some staff, service users may be vulnerable to abuse physically, sexual, emotional, and neglect of care. It is the responsibility of everyone offering care to report these issues to the safeguarding team to make sure these matters are looked into, and solutions found. If you are not sure of what to so once you have identified a problem, reach out to the most senior member of staff on shift to ask for help with this. You could also check the organisation policies on how to go about it.

Gross Misconduct

Gross misconduct is undesired behaviour that is usually determined by a workplace disciplinary committee. It can include things like negligence of service users, theft, physical and sexual violence or serious insubordination.

SUPPORT AVAILABLE TO STAFF

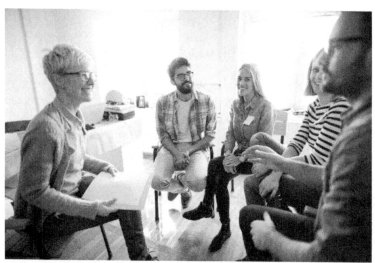

Figure 19: Image showing staff sat together having a bright conversation: Image courtesy of Shutterstock

Working in mental health services is not easy. You are working with vulnerable people and this could begin to show you some of your own vulnerabilities as a person. Sometimes patients could be difficult to relate with causing you to ask yourself existential questions of whether you are cut out for the role. Other times unfortunate events such as passing on of a service user you had developed close relationship with might worsen in mental state or even die and as humans, things like these cloud our minds with grief or some sort of struggle.

Also, personal issues could come into play. For instance, having own struggles with raising young children by yourself, certain shift schedules might not favour you so much. Perhaps you are not having enough rest and this is impacting your productivity, or you are going through a divorce, or loss of a loved one. On the flip side, you could have good things happening but just need guidance on how to handle them for example, you are planning a charity campaign and you need some advice, or you planning a wedding. All, these things have the potential to weigh us down and could massively impact our ability to perform. Such are moments when staff need support. Here are some suggestions of where you could find help.

Fellow staff

It might feel as if your situation is peculiar to you, and that might be true in some ways but in other ways other people working in your workplace could have gone through similar situations before and could offer some peer support

Management

One of the main roles of management is to listen to your grievances and offer the needed support. Talk to the leader of the shift or any other figure of authority you feel comfortable to approach.

Debriefs

These are small meetings organised on the shift to reflect on what happed before, during and after a major incident. For instance, if patients have fought on the ward, or a staff has been assaulted, these sessions are important in establishing if everyone is okay. The brief reflection can evaluate whether a similar thing can be prevented in future and if the team handed it well, and find room for improvement. This is not a time to blame each other but rather see what the positives were, how to uphold these, where the weaknesses were, and how to prevent them from happening again.

Supervision

These are sessions planned by the supervisor as a catch-up session. These are good opportunities to air your frustrations, highlight areas you need support and point out areas you have done well.

Training

Having all the required training for your specific workplace is an excellent way to improve on your confidence. You will feel as if you know what you are doing because you have been trained in it. If at any time you feel you need training in a certain area just ask for it.

Venting

Venting involves letting out your feelings, thoughts and emotions so that people can know. This may be helpful in some situations when done in the right place where there is trust and support.

If done in the wrong setup, it might lead to bad blood among staff, being viewed differently or make it difficult for people to engage with you because they feel inadequate to do so for fear of another vent. Positive venting can occur in places such as the staff room or a spare room involving the aggrieved person and aggravated. A possible third party may be included to support the two to feel safe. Negative venting may occur out in social areas in front of involved parties like service users, or in meetings where the venting is completely unrelated to the matters on the agenda.

REFERENCE LIST

1. AddictionPolicy, A. P. (2022, October 19). *DSM-5 criteria for addiction simplified*. APF. https://www.addictionpolicy.org/post/dsm-5-facts-and-figures

2. Alzheimers.org, Alzheimers. org. (2014). *Drug treatments for alzheimer's disease*. Drug treatments for Alzheimer's disease . https://www.alzheimers.org.uk/sites/default/files/pdf/factsheet_drug_treatments_for_alzheimers_disease.pdf

3. Ameer, M. A., & Saadabadi, A. (2023, August 8). *Neuroleptic medications - statpearls - NCBI bookshelf*. national library of medicine. https://www.ncbi.nlm.nih.gov/books/NBK459150/

4. Anokye, R., Acheampong, E., Budu-Ainooson, A., Obeng, E. I., & Akwasi, A. G. (2018). Prevalence of postpartum depression and interventions utilized for its management. *Annals of General Psychiatry, 17*(1). https://doi.org/10.1186/s12991-018-0188-0

5. APA, A. (2017) *What is exposure therapy?*, *American Psychological Association*. Available at: https://www.apa.org/ptsd-guideline/patients-and-families/exposure-therapy (Accessed: 01 January 2024).

6. APDA, A. (2023, November 21). *Sexual effects of parkinson's: APDA*. American Parkinson Disease Association. https://www.apdaparkinson.org/what-is-parkinsons/symptoms/sexual-effects/#:~:text=Hypersexuality%3A%20While%20occurring%20in%20less,combined%20with%20a%20dopamine%20agonist).

7. Archer, M., Steinvoort, C., Frydrych, V., & Oderda, G. (2016). *Drug class review - utah*. University of Utah College of Pharmacy. https://medicaid.utah.gov/pharmacy/ptcommittee/files/Criteria%20Review%20Documents/2016/2016.05%20Central

%20Nervous%20System%20Stimulants%20Drug%20Clas
s%20Review.pdf

8. Asensio-Aguerri, L., Beato-Fernández, L., Stavraki, M.,
    Rodríguez-Cano, T., Bajo, M., & Díaz, D. (2019).
    Paranoid thinking and wellbeing. the role of doubt in
    pharmacological and metacognitive therapies. *Frontiers in
    Psychology, 10*. https://doi.org/10.3389/fpsyg.2019.02099

9. Babl, A., Gómez Penedo, J. M., Berger, T., Schneider, N.,
    Sachse, R., & Kramer, U. (2022). Change processes in
    psychotherapy for patients presenting with histrionic
    personality disorder. *Clinical Psychology &
    Psychotherapy, 30*(1), 64–72.
    https://doi.org/10.1002/cpp.2769

10. Baldessarini, R.J. and Tondo, L. (2020) 'Suicidal risks in
    12 DSM-5 psychiatric disorders', *Journal of Affective
    Disorders*, 271, pp. 66–73. doi:10.1016/j.jad.2020.03.083.

11. Berman, B. D. (2011, January). *Neuroleptic malignant
    syndrome: A review for neurohospitalists*. The
    Neurohospitalist.
    https://www.ncbi.nlm.nih.gov/pmc/articles/PMC3726098/

12. Bharat, C., Hickman, M., Barbieri, S., & Degenhardt, L.
    (2021). Big Data and predictive modelling for the opioid
    crisis: Existing research and future potential. *The Lancet
    Digital Health, 3*(6). https://doi.org/10.1016/s2589-
    7500(21)00058-3

13. Black, D. W. (2015). The natural history of antisocial
    personality disorder. *The Canadian Journal of Psychiatry,
    60*(7), 309–314.
    https://doi.org/10.1177/070674371506000703

14. BNF, B. (n.d.). *BNF is only available in the UK*. NICE.
    https://bnf.nice.org.uk/drugs/olanzapine/

15. Brager-Larsen, A., Zeiner, P. and Mehlum, L. (2023)
    'DSM-5 non-suicidal self-injury disorder in a clinical
    sample of adolescents with recurrent self-harm behavior',
    Archives of Suicide Research, pp. 1–14.
    doi:10.1080/13811118.2023.2192767.

16. Brown, K. A., Samuel, S., & Patel, D. R. (2017, August
    24). *Pharmacologic management of attention deficit
    hyperactivity disorder in children and adolescents: A
    review for Practitioners*. Translational Pediatrics.
    https://doi.org/10.21037%2Ftp.2017.08.02

17. CDC, C. (2021, August 26). *Trends in nonfatal and fatal
    overdoses involving benzodiazepines - 38 states and the*

District of Columbia, 2019–2020. Centers for Disease Control and Prevention. https://www.cdc.gov/mmwr/volumes/70/wr/mm7034a2.ht m

18. CDC, C. (2022, June 3). *Assessing your weight.* Centers for Disease Control and Prevention. https://www.cdc.gov/healthyweight/assessing/index.html#: ~:text=If%20your%20BMI%20is%2018.5,falls%20within %20the%20obese%20range.

19. Chase, D., Harvey, P.D. and Pogge, D.L. (2020) 'Disruptive mood dysregulation disorder (DMDD) in psychiatric inpatient child admissions: Prevalence among consecutive admissions and in children receiving NOS diagnoses', *Neurology, Psychiatry and Brain Research*, 38, pp. 102–106. doi:10.1016/j.npbr.2020.11.001.

20. Choi-Kain, L. W., Finch, E. F., Masland, S. R., Jenkins, J. A., & Unruh, B. T. (2017, February 3). *What works in the treatment of borderline personality disorder - current behavioral neuroscience reports.* SpringerLink. https://link.springer.com/article/10.1007/s40473-017-0103-z

21. ClevelandClinic, C. (2022) *Prenatal depression: Causes, symptoms & treatment, Cleveland Clinic.* Available at: https://my.clevelandclinic.org/health/diseases/22984-prenatal-depression (Accessed: 31 December 2023).

22. da Silva, M. L., Rocha, R. S., Buheji, M., Jahrami, H., & Cunha, K. da. (2020). A systematic review of the prevalence of anxiety symptoms during coronavirus epidemics. *Journal of Health Psychology, 26*(1), 115–125. https://doi.org/10.1177/1359105320951620

23. Davies, J. A. (1995). Mechanisms of action of Antiepileptic Drugs. *Seizure, 4*(4), 267–271. https://doi.org/10.1016/s1059-1311(95)80003-4

24. DeLisi, M., Drury, A. J., & Elbert, M. J. (2019). The etiology of antisocial personality disorder: The differential roles of adverse childhood experiences and childhood psychopathology. *Comprehensive Psychiatry, 92*, 1–6. https://doi.org/10.1016/j.comppsych.2019.04.001

25. Disney, K. L. (2013). Dependent personality disorder: A critical review. *Clinical Psychology Review, 33*(8), 1184–1196. https://doi.org/10.1016/j.cpr.2013.10.001

26. DrugBank, (n.d.). *Felbamate*. Uses, Interactions, Mechanism of Action | DrugBank Online. https://go.drugbank.com/drugs/DB00949

27. Dunlap, Dr. B. (2023, July 14). *Stages of addiction recovery*. Northern Illinois Recovery Center. https://www.northernillinoisrecovery.com/the-stages-of-addiction-recovery/

28. Eaton, W. W., Bienvenu, O. J., & Miloyan, B. (2018, August). *Specific phobias*. NIH. https://doi.org/10.1016%2FS2215-0366(18)30169-X

29. Eide, T. O., Hjelle, K. M., Sætre, I. U., Solem, S., Olsen, T., Sköld, R. O., Kvale, G., Hansen, B., & Hagen, K. (2023). The Bergen 4-day treatment for panic disorder: Implementation in a rural clinical setting. *BMC Psychiatry*, *23*(1). https://doi.org/10.1186/s12888-023-04812-x

30. Eison, A. S., & Temple, D. L. (1986). Buspirone: Review of its pharmacology and current perspectives on its mechanism of action. *The American Journal of Medicine*, *80*(3), 1–9. https://doi.org/10.1016/0002-9343(86)90325-6

31. Ettinger, U., Meyhöfer, I., Steffens, M., Wagner, M., & Koutsouleris, N. (2014). Genetics, cognition, and neurobiology of schizotypal personality: A review of the overlap with schizophrenia. *Frontiers in Psychiatry*, *5*. https://doi.org/10.3389/fpsyt.2014.00018

32. Fariba, K. A., Madhanagopal, N., & Gupta, V. (2022, June 9). *Schizoid personality disorder - statpearls - NCBI bookshelf*. National Library of medicine . https://www.ncbi.nlm.nih.gov/books/NBK559234/

33. Farzam, K., Faizy, R. M., & Saadabadi, A. (2023, July). *Stimulants - statpearls - NCBI bookshelf*. NIH. https://www.ncbi.nlm.nih.gov/books/NBK539896/

34. Forstner, A. J., Awasthi, S., Wolf, C., Maron, E., Erhardt, A., Czamara, D., Eriksson, E., Lavebratt, C., Allgulander, C., Friedrich, N., Becker, J., Hecker, J., Rambau, S., Conrad, R., Geiser, F., McMahon, F. J., Moebus, S., Hess, T., Buerfent, B. C., … Schumacher, J. (2019, November 11). *Genome-wide association study of panic disorder reveals genetic overlap with neuroticism and Depression*. Nature News. https://www.nature.com/articles/s41380-019-0590-2

35. Freeman, A.J. *et al.* (2016) 'Disruptive mood dysregulation disorder in a community mental health clinic: Prevalence, comorbidity and correlates', *Journal of*

Child and Adolescent Psychopharmacology, 26(2), pp. 123–130. doi:10.1089/cap.2015.0061.
36. Gaebel, W., & Zielasek, J. (2015). Focus on psychosis. *Dialogues in Clinical Neuroscience*, *17*(1), 9–18. https://doi.org/10.31887/dcns.2015.17.1/wgaebel
37. Gancher, S. (2010). Benzodiazepines and movement disorders. *Encyclopedia of Movement Disorders*, 130–134. https://doi.org/10.1016/b978-0-12-374105-9.00306-3
38. Gecaite-Stonciene, J., Lochner, C., Marincowitz, C., Fineberg, N. A., & Stein, D. J. (2021, February 19). *Obsessive-compulsive (anankastic) personality disorder in the ICD-11: A scoping review.* Frontiers. https://www.frontiersin.org/articles/10.3389/fpsyt.2021.64 6030/full
39. Gifford, T. (2022, July 18). *Build your hedge of protection against disease with macro counting.* Stay Fit Mom. https://stayfitmom.com/build-your-hedge-of-protection-against-disease-with-macro-counting/
40. Henderson, D. C., Fan, X., Copeland, P. M., Sharma, B., Borba, C. P., Boxill, R., Freudenreich, O., Cather, C., Evins, A. E., & Goff, D. C. (2009, April). *Aripiprazole added to overweight and obese olanzapine-treated schizophrenia patients.* Journal of clinical psychopharmacology. https://www.ncbi.nlm.nih.gov/pmc/articles/PMC4311767/ #:~:text=Another%20study%20found%20that%2094,to%2 0olanzapine%20therapy%204%2C5.
41. Howard E. LeWine, M. (2022, March 10). *Major depression.* Harvard Health. https://www.health.harvard.edu/a_to_z/major-depression-a-to-z
42. HSC, H. (n.d.). *Basic principles.* Basic Principles | PHA Infection Control. https://www.niinfectioncontrolmanual.net/basic-principles
43. Jain, A., & Mitra, P. (2023, February). *Bipolar disorder - statpearls - NCBI bookshelf.* NIH. https://www.ncbi.nlm.nih.gov/books/NBK558998/
44. Jett, D. A. (1998). Central cholinergic neurobiology. *Handbook of Developmental Neurotoxicology*, 257–274. https://doi.org/10.1016/b978-012648860-9.50018-2
45. JHM, J. (2023, November 3). *Major depression.* Johns Hopkins Medicine.

https://www.hopkinsmedicine.org/health/conditions-and-diseases/major-depression
46. JohnsHopkinsMedicine, J. (no date) *Seasonal affective disorder, Johns Hopkins Medicine*. Available at: https://www.hopkinsmedicine.org/health/conditions-and-diseases/seasonal-affective-disorder#:~:text=Seasonal%20affective%20disorder%2C%20or%20SAD,antidepressants%20can%20help%20treat%20SAD. (Accessed: 31 December 2023).
47. Jung, Y., & Namkoong, K. (2014). Alcohol. *Handbook of Clinical Neurology*, 115–121. https://doi.org/10.1016/b978-0-444-62619-6.00007-0
48. Kang, M., Galuska, M., & Ghassemzadeh, S. (2023, June 26). *Benzodiazepine toxicity - statpearls - NCBI bookshelf*. NIH. https://www.ncbi.nlm.nih.gov/books/NBK482238/
49. King, W. (n.d.). *Abnormal psychology*. Lumen. https://courses.lumenlearning.com/wm-abnormalpsych/chapter/pica/
50. Kiohan, E. (2023, June 22). *Therapy for narcissistic personality disorder - talkspace*. Mental Health Conditions. https://www.talkspace.com/mental-health/conditions/narcissistic-personality-disorder/therapy-treatment-types/
51. Koenen, K. C., Ratanatharathorn, A., Ng, L., McLaughlin, K. A., Bromet, E. J., Stein, D. J., Karam, E. G., Ruscio, A. M., Benjet, C., Scott, K., Atwoli, L., Petukhova, M., Lim, C. C. W., Aguilar-Gaxiola, S., Al-Hamzawi, A., Alonso, J., Bunting, B., Ciutan, M., Girolamo, G. de, … Kessler, R. C. (2017, April 7). *Posttraumatic stress disorder in the World Mental Health Surveys: Psychological Medicine*. Cambridge Core. https://doi.org/10.1017%2FS0033291717000708
52. Kouli, A., Torsney, K.M. and Kuan., W.-L. (2018) *Parkinson's disease: Etiology, neuropathology, and pathogenesis, National library of medicine* . Available at: https://www.ncbi.nlm.nih.gov/books/NBK536722/ (Accessed: 29 December 2023).
53. Lake, S., Socías, M. E., & Milloy, M.-J. (2020). Evidence shows that cannabis has fewer relative harms than opioids. *Canadian Medical Association Journal*, *192*(7). https://doi.org/10.1503/cmaj.74120
54. Lee, E., & Jang, M. H. (2021, April 7). *The influence of body image, insight, and mental health confidence on*

medication adherence in young adult women with mental disorders. MDPI. https://doi.org/10.3390%2Fijerph18083866

55. Lee, Y.-L., Tien, Y., Bai, Y.-S., Lin, C.-K., Yin, C.-S., Chung, C.-H., Sun, C.-A., Huang, S.-H., Huang, Y.-C., Chien, W.-C., Kang, C.-Y., & Wu, G.-J. (2022, April 23). *Association of postpartum depression with maternal suicide: A nationwide population-based study.* MDPI. https://doi.org/10.3390%2Fijerph19095118

56. Lieberman, J. A. (2004). *Managing anticholinergic side effects.* Primary care companion to the Journal of clinical psychiatry. https://www.ncbi.nlm.nih.gov/pmc/articles/PMC487008/#:~:text=Typical%20symptoms%20include%20dry%20mouth,decreased%20sweating%20(Table%201).

57. Lohia, A., & McKenzie, J. (2023, July 24). *Neuroanatomy, pyramidal tract lesions - statpearls - NCBI bookshelf.* NIH. https://www.ncbi.nlm.nih.gov/books/NBK540976/

58. Mansoor, M., McNeil, R., Fleming, T., Barker, A., Vakharia, S., Sue, K., & Ivsins, A. (2022). Characterizing stimulant overdose: A qualitative study on perceptions and experiences of "overamping." *International Journal of Drug Policy, 102,* 103592. https://doi.org/10.1016/j.drugpo.2022.103592

59. Mayoclinic, M. (2022, April 28). *Relaxation techniques: Try these steps to reduce stress.* Mayo Clinic. https://www.mayoclinic.org/healthy-lifestyle/stress-management/in-depth/relaxation-technique/art-20045368

60. MayoClinic, M. (2023) *Self-injury/cutting, Mayo Clinic.* Available at: https://www.mayoclinic.org/diseases-conditions/self-injury/diagnosis-treatment/drc-20350956 (Accessed: 01 January 2024).

61. Mayoclinic, M. (2023, August 30). *How alzheimer's drugs help manage symptoms.* Mayo Clinic. https://www.mayoclinic.org/diseases-conditions/alzheimers-disease/in-depth/alzheimers/art-20048103#:~:text=Common%20side%20effects%20include%20dizziness,%2C%20dizziness%2C%20nausea%20and%20diarrhea.

62. Mind, M. (2020). *What are mood stabilisers?* https://www.mind.org.uk/information-support/drugs-and-treatments/lithium-and-other-mood-stabilisers/about-mood-stabilisers/

63. Mind, M. (n.d.). *Side effects of antidepressants.* https://www.mind.org.uk/information-support/drugs-and-treatments/antidepressants/side-effects-of-antidepressants/
64. Moitra, M., Owens, S., Hailemariam, M., Wilson, K., Mensa-Kwao, A., Gonese, G., Kamamia, C., White, B., Young, D., & Collins , P. (2023, May 31). *Global Mental Health: Where we are and where we are going.* Current psychiatry reports. https://pubmed.ncbi.nlm.nih.gov/37256471/
65. Montgomery, E. (2016) *The Science of Music therapy, Peterson Family Foundation.* Available at: https://petersonfamilyfoundation.org/music-therapy/science-music-therapy/ (Accessed: 01 January 2024).
66. Moore, M. (2022) *The ultimate list of phobias, Psych Central.* Available at: https://psychcentral.com/disorders/list-of-phobias#summary (Accessed: 31 December 2023).
67. Moutier, C. (2023) *Suicidal behavior - psychiatric disorders, MSD Manual Professional Edition.* Available at: https://www.msdmanuals.com/en-gb/professional/psychiatric-disorders/suicidal-behavior-and-self-injury/suicidal-behavior#:~:text=Suicidal%20behavior%20encompasses%20a%20spectrum,%2C%20considering%2C%20or%20planning%20suicide. (Accessed: 01 January 2024).
68. Mughal, S., Azhar, Y., & Siddiqui, W. (2022, October). *Postpartum depression - statpearls - NCBI bookshelf.* Postpartum Depression. https://www.ncbi.nlm.nih.gov/books/NBK519070/
69. Mutanana, N., Tsvere, M., & Chiweshe, M. K. (2020). *General side effects and challenges associated with anti-epilepsy medication: A review of related literature.* African Journal of Primary Health Care & Family Medicine. https://doi.org/10.4102%2Fphcfm.v12i1.2162
70. Nasser, Y. A., Muco, E., & Alsaad, A. J. (2023, June). *Pica - StatPearls - NCBI Bookshelf.* NIH. https://www.ncbi.nlm.nih.gov/books/NBK532242/
71. Nath, M., & Gupta, V. (2023, April). *Mood stabilizers - statpearls - NCBI bookshelf.* NIH. https://www.ncbi.nlm.nih.gov/books/NBK556141/
72. NCBI, N. (no date) *Aromatherapy with essential oils (PDQ®): Health Professional Version, National Center*

for Biotechnology Information. Available at: https://pubmed.ncbi.nlm.nih.gov/26389313/ (Accessed: 01 January 2024).

73. NHS, N. (2022). *Signs of autism in children*. NHS choices. https://www.nhs.uk/conditions/autism/signs/children/
74. NHS, N. (2023, December 21). *Obsessive-compulsive disorder (OCD)*. Mayo Clinic. https://www.mayoclinic.org/diseases-conditions/obsessive-compulsive-disorder/symptoms-causes/syc-20354432
75. NHS, N. (n.d.). *Bipolar disorder*. NHS choices. https://www.nhs.uk/mental-health/conditions/bipolar-disorder/
76. NIH, N. (2021). *What are the treatments for autism?*. Eunice Kennedy Shriver National Institute of Child Health and Human Development. https://www.nichd.nih.gov/health/topics/autism/conditioninfo/treatments
77. NIH, N. (n.d.-a). *How is alzheimer's disease treated?* National Institute on Aging. https://www.nia.nih.gov/health/alzheimers-treatment/how-alzheimers-disease-treated#:~:text=Galantamine%2C%20rivastigmine%2C%20and%20donepezil%20are,some%20cognitive%20and%20behavioral%20symptoms.
78. NIH, N. (n.d.-b). *Understanding psychosis*. National Institute of Mental Health. https://www.nimh.nih.gov/health/publications/understanding-psychosis
79. NIH, N. (no date a) *Disruptive mood dysregulation disorder: The basics, National Institute of Mental Health*. Available at: https://www.nimh.nih.gov/health/publications/disruptive-mood-dysregulation-disorder#:~:text=What%20is%20disruptive%20mood%20dysregulation,.%E2%80%9D%20DMDD%20symptoms%20are%20severe. (Accessed: 31 December 2023).
80. NIH, N. (no date b) *Relaxation techniques for health, National Center for Complementary and Integrative Health*. Available at: https://www.nccih.nih.gov/health/relaxation-techniques-what-you-need-to-know#:~:text=Relaxation%20techniques%20are%20practi

ces%20to,opposite%20of%20the%20stress%20response. (Accessed: 01 January 2024).

81. NIH, N. (no date c) *Warning signs of suicide, National Institute of Mental Health*. Available at: https://www.nimh.nih.gov/health/publications/warning-signs-of-suicide (Accessed: 01 January 2024).

82. Oquendo, M.A. and Baca-Garcia, E. (2014) 'Suicidal behavior disorder as a diagnostic entity in the DSM-5 classification system: Advantages outweigh limitations', *World Psychiatry*, 13(2), pp. 128–130. doi:10.1002/wps.20116.

83. Patel, J., & Marwaha, R. (2023, July 24). *Akathisia*. National Center for Biotechnology Information. https://pubmed.ncbi.nlm.nih.gov/30137828/

84. Pelek, A. (2022) *Phobias: DSM-5, types, diagnosis and treatment - psycom*, MedCentral. Available at: https://www.medcentral.com/behavioral-mental/anxiety/assessment-diagnosis-adherence-phobia (Accessed: 31 December 2023).

85. Petre, A. (2022, May 18). *Learn about 6 common types of eating disorders and their symptoms*. Healthline. https://www.healthline.com/nutrition/common-eating-disorders#-6.-Avoidant/restrictive-food-intake-disorder

86. Pittenger, C., Kelmendi, B., Bloch, M., Krystal, J. H., & Coric, V. (2005, November). *Clinical treatment of obsessive compulsive disorder*. Psychiatry (Edgmont (Pa. : Township)). https://www.ncbi.nlm.nih.gov/pmc/articles/PMC2993523/#:~:text=Behavioral%20Treatment%20of%20OCD&text=Exposure%20and%20response%20prevention%20(ERP,engaging%20in%20their%20usual%20compulsions.

87. Pope, C. (2023, April). *List of atypical antipsychotics + uses, types & side effects*. Drugs.com. https://www.drugs.com/drug-class/atypical-antipsychotics.html#

88. Pratt, S. (n.d.). *Histrionic personality disorder symptoms, causes & treatment*. Sheppard Pratt. https://www.sheppardpratt.org/knowledge-center/condition/histrionic-personality-disorder/#:~:text=Histrionic%20Personality%20Disorder%20Treatment&text=Medication%3A%20There%20is%20no%20medication,effective%20in%20treating%20this%20disorder.

89. Prochaska, J. O., & Velicer, W. F. (1997). The transtheoretical model of Health Behavior Change. *American Journal of Health Promotion, 12*(1), 38–48. https://doi.org/10.4278/0890-1171-12.1.38

90. professional, C. C. medical. (n.d.). *Sleep disorders: Conditions that prevent you from getting restful sleep.* Cleveland Clinic. https://my.clevelandclinic.org/health/diseases/11429-sleep-disorders

91. PsychDB, P. (2021, March 6). *Introduction to mood stabilizers and anticonvulsants.* https://www.psychdb.com/meds/mood-stabilizers-anticonvulsants/home#:~:text=not%20exacerbate%20symptoms.-,Mechanism%20of%20Action,channels%20or%20intracellular%20signalling%20pathways.

92. RCH, R. (n.d.). *The Royal Children's hospital melbourne.* The Royal Children's Hospital Melbourne. https://www.rch.org.au/neurology/patient_information/antiepileptic_medications/#:~:text=Some%20mild%20side%20effects%20are,irritability%2C%20anxiety%20or%20mood%20changes.

93. Richard, A., Rohrmann, S., Pestoni, G., Strippoli, M.-P. F., Lasserre, A., Marques-Vidal, P., Preisig, M., & Vandeleur, C. L. (2022). Associations between anxiety disorders and diet quality in a Swiss cohort study. *Comprehensive Psychiatry, 118*, 152344. https://doi.org/10.1016/j.comppsych.2022.152344

94. Schimelpfening, N. (2022, November 12). *The 5 major types of antidepressants.* Verywell Mind. https://www.verywellmind.com/what-are-the-major-classes-of-antidepressants-1065086

95. Sekhon, S., & Gupta, V. (2023, May 8). *Mood disorder - statpearls - NCBI bookshelf.* National Library of Medicine. https://www.ncbi.nlm.nih.gov/books/NBK558911/

96. Shacknai, G. (2020) *The science behind Aromatherapy - Shondaland, shondaland.* Available at: https://www.shondaland.com/live/body/a34330756/the-science-behind-aromatherapy/ (Accessed: 01 January 2024).

97. Stroup , T. S., & Gray, N. (2018, September). *Management of common adverse effects of antipsychotic medications ...* world psychiatry.

https://www.researchgate.net/publication/327512873_Man
agement_of_common_adverse_effects_of_antipsychotic_
medications_World_Psychiatry

98. Subramaniam, M., Soh, P., Vaingankar, J. A., Picco, L., &
Chong, S. A. (2013, April 12). *Quality of life in obsessive-
compulsive disorder: Impact of the disorder and of
treatment - CNS drugs*. SpringerLink.
https://link.springer.com/article/10.1007/s40263-013-
0056-z

99. Tadvi, N. (2016, May 2). *Antiepileptics*. PPT.
https://www.slideshare.net/nasertadvi/antiepileptics-
61566897

100. Trần, V., Szabó, Á., Ward, C., & Jose, P. E. (2023). To
vent or not to vent? the impact of venting on psychological
symptoms varies by levels of social support. *International
Journal of Intercultural Relations*, *92*, 101750.
https://doi.org/10.1016/j.ijintrel.2022.101750

101. Vasan, S., & Padhy, R. K. (2023, April). *Tardive
dyskinesia*. National Center for Biotechnology
Information. https://pubmed.ncbi.nlm.nih.gov/28846278/

102. Vyas, A., & Khan, M. (2016). Paranoid personality
disorder. *American Journal of Psychiatry Residents'
Journal*, *11*(1), 9–11. https://doi.org/10.1176/appi.ajp-
rj.2016.110103

103. Wahass, S. H. (2005, May). *The role of psychologists in
Health Care Delivery*. Journal of family & community
medicine.
https://www.ncbi.nlm.nih.gov/pmc/articles/PMC3410123/

104. WebMD, W. (2023) *EMDR therapy (Eye Movement
Desensitization & reprocessing)*, *WebMD*. Available at:
https://www.webmd.com/mental-health/emdr-what-is-it
(Accessed: 01 January 2024).

105. Whitten, C. (2023, January 9). *Anxiolytic medications:
Types and side effects*. WebMD.
https://www.webmd.com/anxiety-panic/what-are-
anxiolytics

106. WHO, W. (2012). *Role of anticholinergic medications in
patients requiring long-term antipsychotic treatment for
psychotic disorders*. World Health Organization.
https://www.who.int/teams/mental-health-and-substance-
use/treatment-care/mental-health-gap-action-
programme/evidence-centre/psychosis-and-bipolar-
disorders/role-of-anticholinergic-medications-in-patients-

requiring-long-term-antipsychotic-treatment-for-psychotic-disorders

107. Williams , B. C. (2022, June 9). *Marijuana Overdose: Cannabis overdose treatment, signs, & symptoms.* The Recovery Village Drug and Alcohol Rehab. https://www.therecoveryvillage.com/marijuana-addiction/marijuana-overdose/

108. Wittchen, H.-U. (2002). Generalized anxiety disorder: Prevalence, burden, and cost to society. *Depression and Anxiety, 16*(4), 162–171. https://doi.org/10.1002/da.10065

109. Yurdagül, C., Kircaburun, K., Emirtekin, E., Wang, P., & Griffiths, M. D. (2022, August 15). *Psychopathological consequences related to problematic Instagram use among adolescents: The mediating role of body image dissatisfaction and moderating role of gender - international journal of mental health and addiction.* SpringerLink. https://link.springer.com/article/10.1007/s11469-019-00071-8

110. Zetterqvist, M. *et al.* (2020) 'Nonsuicidal self-injury disorder in adolescents: Clinical utility of the diagnosis using the clinical assessment of nonsuicidal self-injury disorder index', *Frontiers in Psychiatry*, 11. doi:10.3389/fpsyt.2020.00008.

111. Zimmerman, M. (2023, December 8). *Avoidant personality disorder (AVPD) - psychiatric disorders.* MSD Manual Professional Edition. https://www.msdmanuals.com/en-gb/professional/psychiatric-disorders/personality-disorders/avoidant-personality-disorder-avpd

Printed in Great Britain
by Amazon

45167298R00069